HowExpert Presents

Kickboxing 101

A Beginner's Guide To Kickboxing For Self Defense, Fitness, and Fun

HowExpert with Nathan DeMetz

For more tips related to this topic, visit HowExpert.com/kickboxing.

Recommended Resources

- HowExpert.com – Quick 'How To' Guides on All Topics from A to Z by Everyday Experts.
- HowExpert.com/free – Free HowExpert Email Newsletter.
- HowExpert.com/books – HowExpert Books
- HowExpert.com/courses – HowExpert Courses
- HowExpert.com/clothing – HowExpert Clothing
- HowExpert.com/membership – HowExpert Membership Site
- HowExpert.com/affiliates – HowExpert Affiliate Program
- HowExpert.com/writers – Write About Your #1 Passion/Knowledge/Expertise & Become a HowExpert Author.
- HowExpert.com/resources – Additional HowExpert Recommended Resources
- YouTube.com/HowExpert – Subscribe to HowExpert YouTube.
- Instagram.com/HowExpert – Follow HowExpert on Instagram.
- Facebook.com/HowExpert – Follow HowExpert on Facebook.

Table of Contents

Introduction

What Is Kickboxing?

Kickboxing is a stand-up form of striking. It consists of a variety of attacks, but is commonly known for strikes with the hands and legs (punches and kicks). This is only a small part of kickboxing, however, as the form of combat includes knee strikes, elbow strikes, open palm techniques, and many other stand-up attacks.

Many people, maybe even you, envision kickboxing as the atypical straight punches (the jab and cross) as well as the atypical roundhouse kick, which is more often simply referred to as a round kick. This is a beginning point for kickboxing, but even a straight punch or a round kick are not as simple as they first seem. For example, there are different versions of the round kick, or roundhouse kick. A round kick in Tae Kwon Do is different from a round kick in Muay Thai. The same can be said for other striking forms of martial arts as well.

Kickboxing is a well-rounded form of martial arts that is not in itself a traditional martial art. Kickboxing, as I know it, is a culmination of many striking martial arts. Depending on where a person has trained, and with whom, the styles they are associated with may differ. For me, I primarily use Boxing and Muay Thai, while incorporating some techniques from other arts. For an associate of mine, their base is in Tae Kwon Do with supplemental training in boxing and Muay Thai.

The more you search and talk with different people or groups, the more you will see variety in what "kickboxing" is for each person.

The History of The Art

Just as kickboxing is diverse and hard to define in simple terms, so is the history of the art. Various forms of stand-up striking martial arts date back to ancient times. You can be sure that some forms, if we were able to truly follow them all the way back in time, predate historical records.

Muay Thai predates the 19th century and originates in Thailand. The style is the successor of Muay Boran. Other variations of Muay Thai and Muay Boran exist. Styles that predate Muay Boran and Muay Thai are argued to be basis for Muay Boran and other arts influenced, or are influenced by, Muay Boran.

Records on Karate vary depending on the style, historian, and other factors. According to some accounts, Karate can be traced back to Zen Buddhism in Western India with an inception date of around 1400 years ago. Others trace the history of karate back to the 19th century, but state possible earlier beginnings.

My point is, when you look at the details of and think about kickboxing, do not dial it down to one area or set of skills. Thinks of it as a larger spectrum of skills and disciplines that can be put to together in nearly infinite ways. Appreciate where the art has come from and where it will go.

What Will You Learn in This Manual?

The point of this manual is to impart on you as much of the basics as I can within the limited amount of space available. This will include proper stance, attacks, movement, and more. The idea is to provide you with a well-rounded, working knowledge that you can perfect on your own or with a partner, from home or in a class environment, as a primary learning tool or as a supplement to other learning. Specific chapters covered in this manual will be:

Chapter 1: Stance and movement: This chapter will cover the appropriate foot stance and hand positioning, as well as variations. Movement will also be covered and include lateral, side, and pivoting.

Chapter 2: Defense – blocking and evasion: This chapter will show you how to evade punches using traditional boxing movements, such as the slip or bob-n-weave.

Chapter 3: Attacking with punches: In this chapter, you will learn to attack with punches, such as the jab, cross, hook, and uppercut, as well as other variations.

Chapter 4: Basic elbow and knee attacks: Knees and elbows will be discussed in this chapter with multiple variations of both being covered. The round elbow, downward elbow, basic knee, and knee with head grab are some techniques you will learn.

Chapter 5: Basic kick attacks: Kicks of various types will be taught in this chapter. The kicks will be basic and include the rear-leg round kick, teep (push kick), and the front-leg round kick. Defensive maneuvers, such as the shielding and kick checking will be included as well.

Chapter 6: Putting it together: This chapter will show you how to put everything you learned together. It will outline potential combos and more.

Safety First

Before we move on, I want to emphasize the importance of safety. Safety is always an important issue to take into consideration. When performing martial arts, or any type of strenuous activity, injuries can occur. To minimize this, precautions should be taken. Always attempt to perform movement in a controlled manner. When working with a partner, be sure both of you understand what training will be covered. Decide what level of power and intensity will be used. Always practice in an area that is safe for training and use the necessary protective gear. This includes, but is not limited to, head gear, a mouth guard, gloves, and striking pads.

Chapter 1: Stance and Movement

Before learning any other aspect of kickboxing, you must first know how to stand and how to move. We will begin with stance. There are two basic stances for any type of striking based form of combat. They are the **Orthodox** and **Southpaw** stance.

The Orthodox stance is the positioning that a right-handed person generally uses. This puts their right hand, or power hand, and their right foot in the rear position. People who use the Southpaw stance are the exact opposite. Their left hand is in the rear position as is their left foot.

Stances can vary greatly in both the Southpaw and Orthodox stances. Foot positioning, knee bend, and other factors are aspects of stance. The following series of photos will outline some of the variations for foot positioning and knee bend in the Orthodox and Southpaw stances.

Orthodox Stance

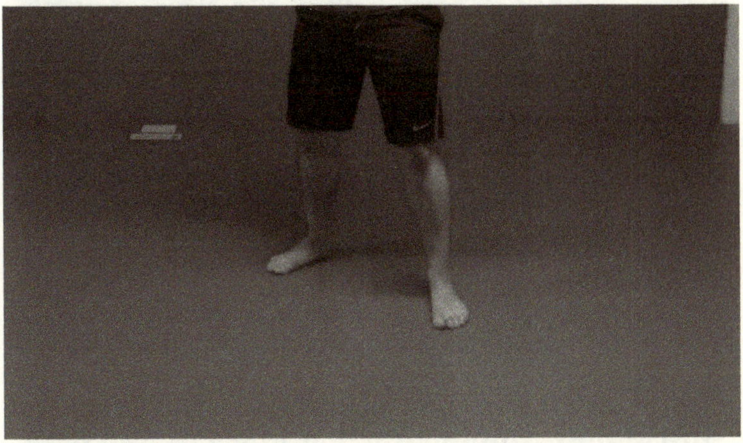

Figure 1: This is the basic kickboxing stance that I use when throwing strikes. I suggest you use this same stance. It can vary slightly to accommodate your body type and to ensure comfort in movement. This stance is ideal for throwing quick and powerful strikes. I use a slightly deeper knee bend when I am evading certain strikes or throwing certain strikes. You will notice this as you work through the manual.

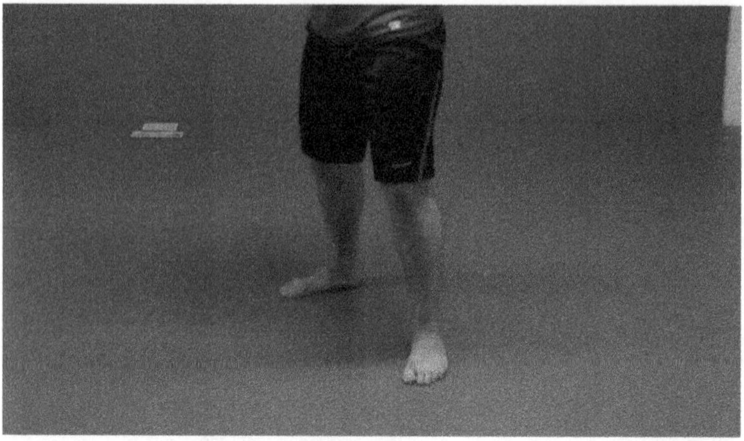

Figure 2: This is the basic stance that I use for movement. Having my feet more in line with each other allows me to push off the back foot in order to move forward. This same idea applies to other movement as well. I will go over movement further in this chapter.

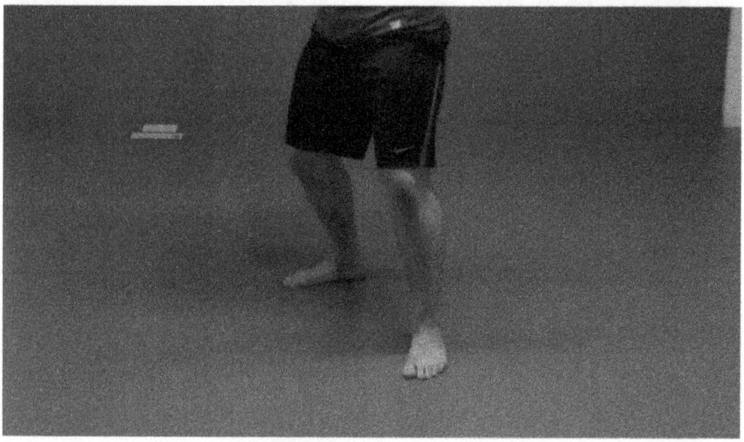

Figure 3: This is an example of the deeper knee bend I will use.

Southpaw Stance

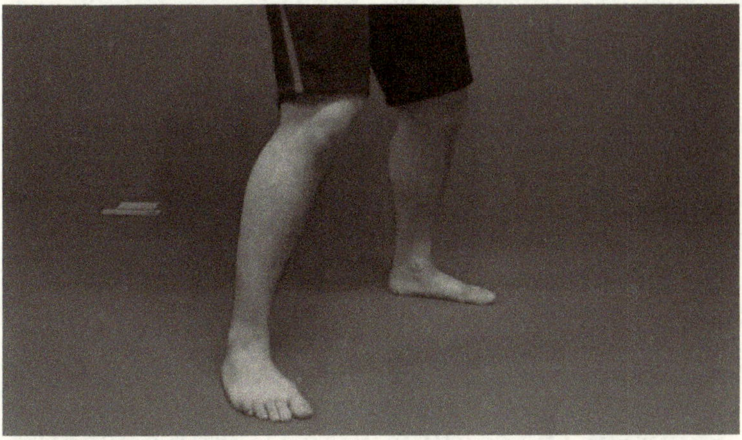

Figure 4: This is a foot shot of the southpaw stance. The stance is a reverse of the orthodox stance. It is used by a person who is left handed. The southpaw fighter has their left foot back and their right foot forward.

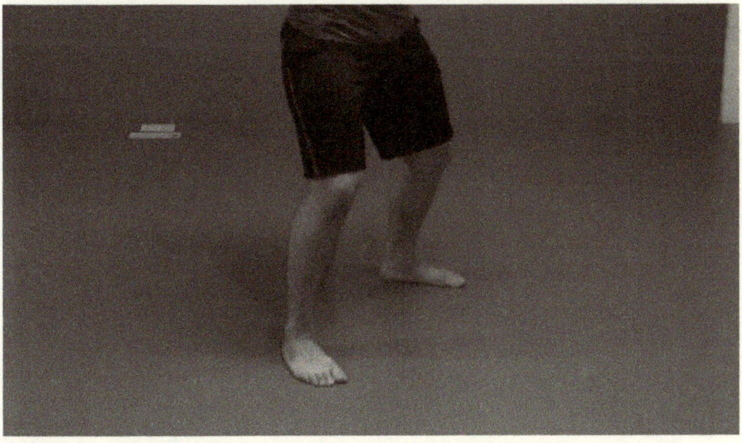

Figure 5: This is the southpaw stance with the deeper knee bend.

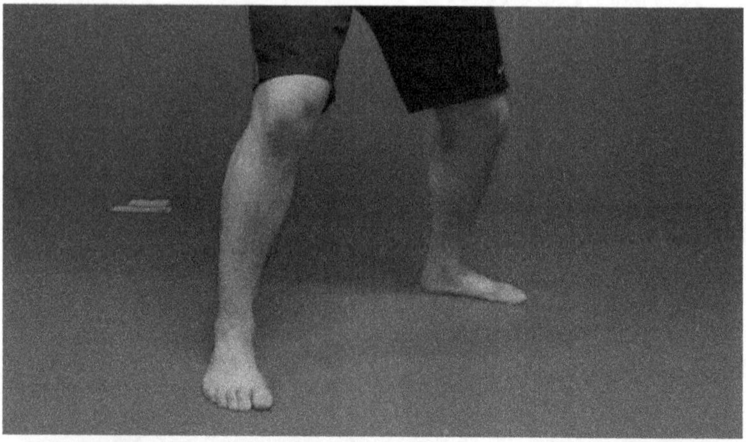

Figure 6: The southpaw stance with a slightly wider stance used for seating down on punches. This can be used in both the southpaw and orthodox stances. The wider stance can create greater power generation. This will be discussed more later.

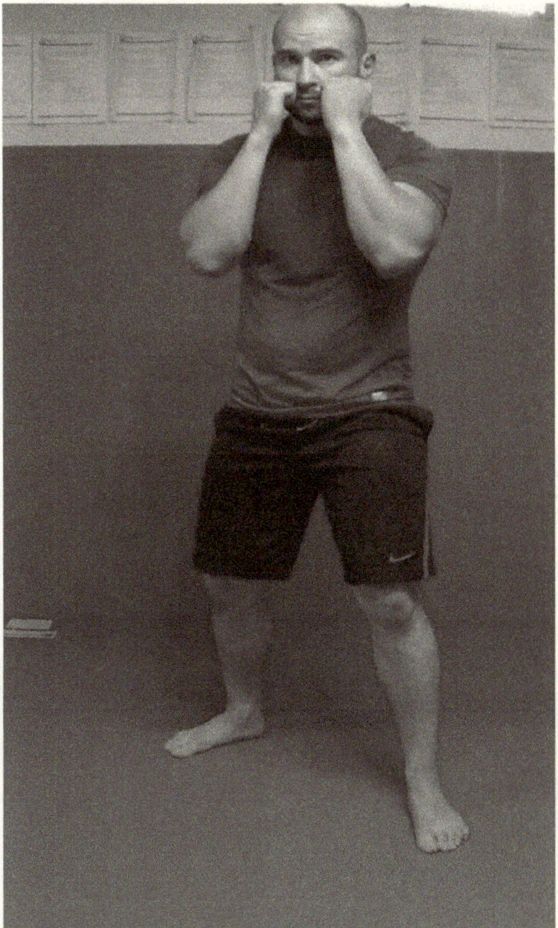

Figure 7: In this image, the orthodox stance is displayed in full body view. The foot stance is slightly wider which is used for seating down on punches. This is more of a power stance than a movement stance. Notice that the hands are kept high and close to the face. Notice the slight bend in the knees.

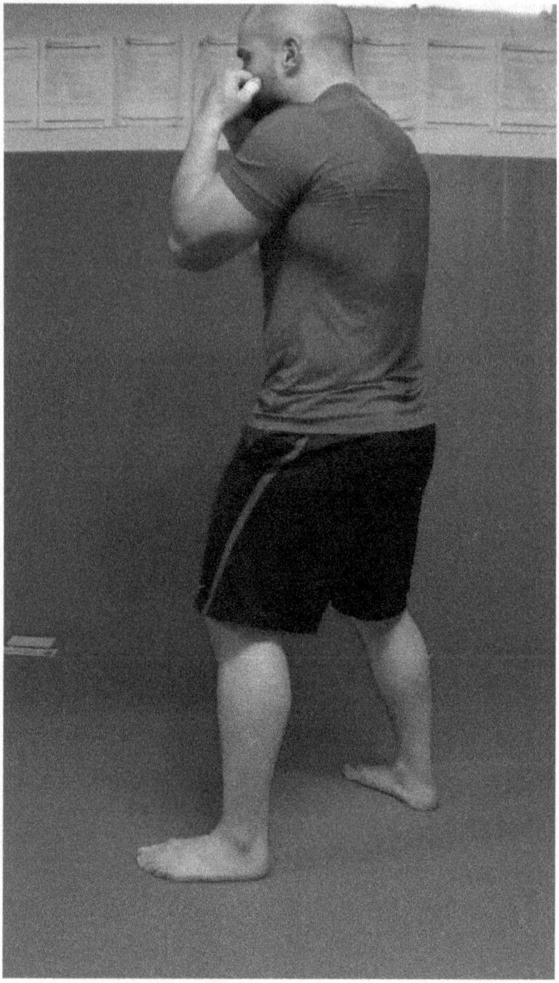

Figure 8: This a left-side view of the stance form figure 7. Again, notice the slight knee bend, high and tight guard, and the slightly wider stance.

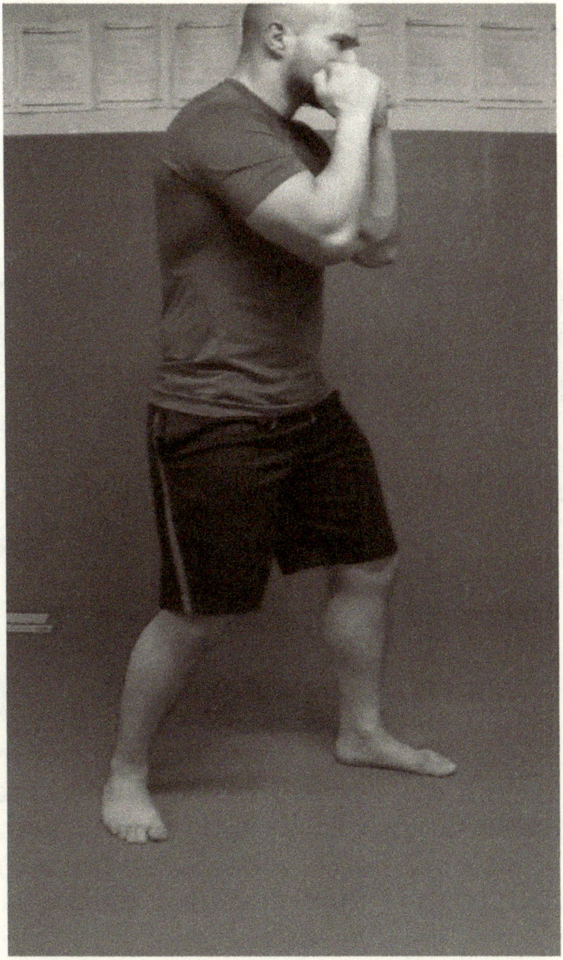

Figure 9: The right-side view of figure 7. From this angle, you can see how the head, elbows, knees, and body align. You can see the solidity of the foot stance.

The preceding stances referenced and imaged are the primary stances you will use in conjunction with this manual. There is one other stance you will also use called the side stance.

Side Stance

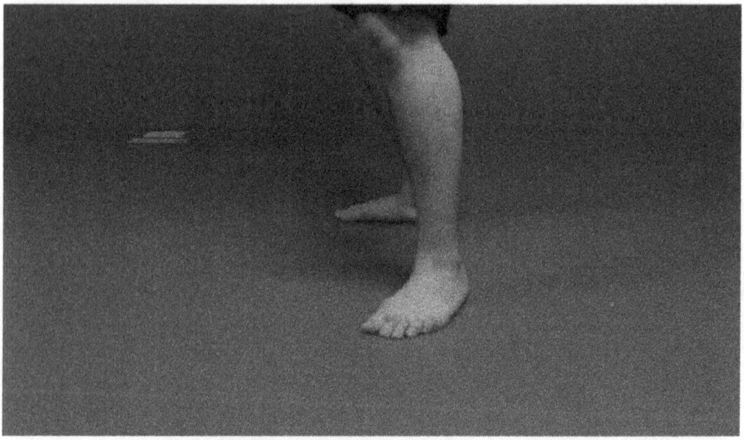

Figure 10: The side stance looks just how it sounds. You will stand with your body faced to the side with your head looking forward. The foot position is front to back, meaning one is in front of the other, standing on the same line.

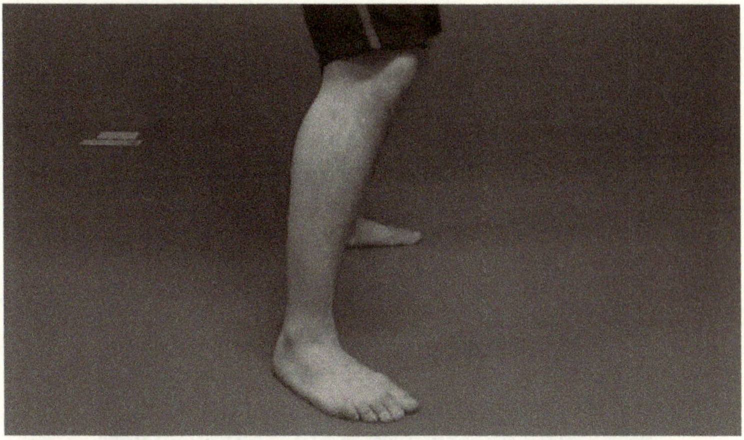

Figure 11: The side stance works from both sides and is used for certain kicking strikes. A sidekick and a turning back kick (spinning back kick) are two kicks thrown from this position.

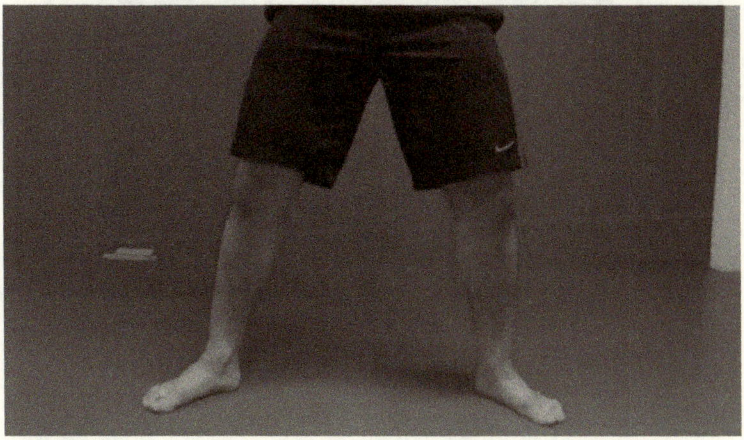

Figure 12: The side view of the side stance. Notice the positioning of the feet and the angle of the feet.

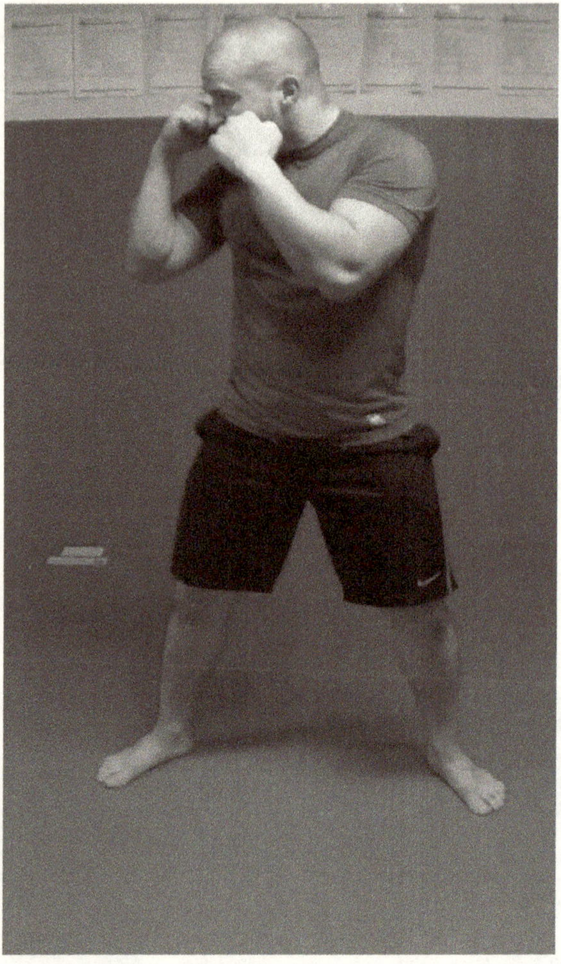

Figure 13: Full body view of the side stance. Your hands are still held high and the face looks forward toward your opponent.

Flat Footed vs. Ball Footing

In boxing and kickboxing, there are two basic types of footing. These refer to the way the bottoms of your feet contact the ground. The first is **standing flatfooted** while the second is **standing ball footed**. Standing flatfooted means standing with your entire foot touching the ground. This is the way most people stand every day and it is the way you want to stand when throwing certain strikes from the upper body.

Standing on the balls of your feet (ball footed) refers to standing with the heels of your feet slightly off the ground with your weight supported by the balls of your feet. The balls of your feet are the front part of the foot behind the toes. This footing is used for movement and for throwing certain strikes from the lower body.

Standing Ball Footed

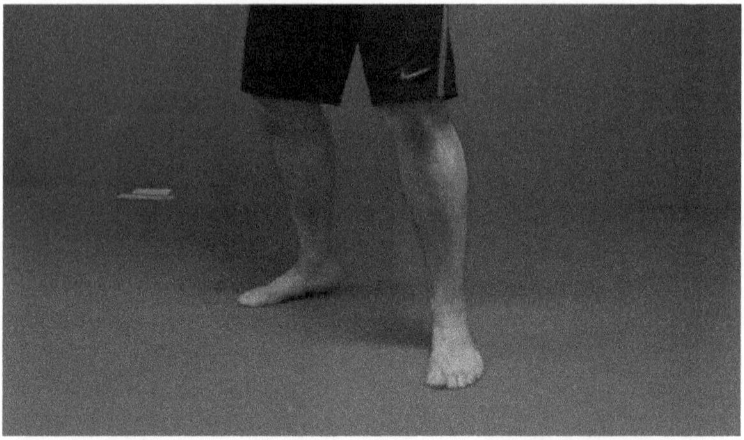

Figure 14: It may be a little hard to see, but I am standing ball footed in this image. I am only slightly lifted. It does not need to be an extreme lift but rather just enough to distribute weight to the balls of the feet.

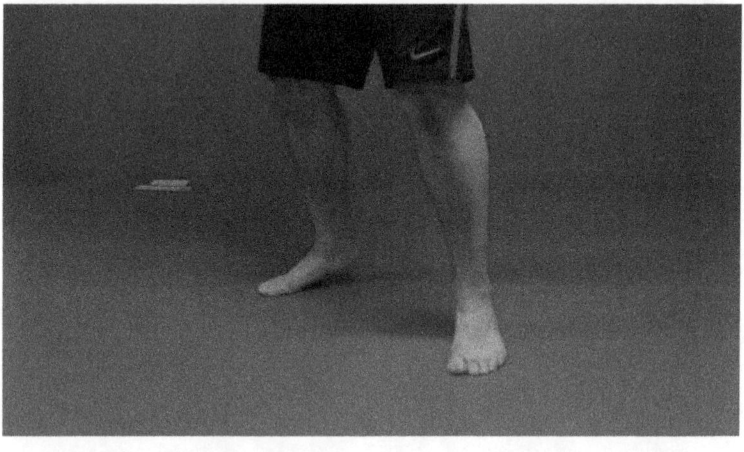

Figure 15: Here I am again standing ball footed although it is exaggerated. Being this

high on the balls of the feet when stationary is unnecessary. Only in mid-motion will you be elevated this high on the balls of the feet. At a standstill, this leads to an unbalanced stance.

Standing Flat Footed

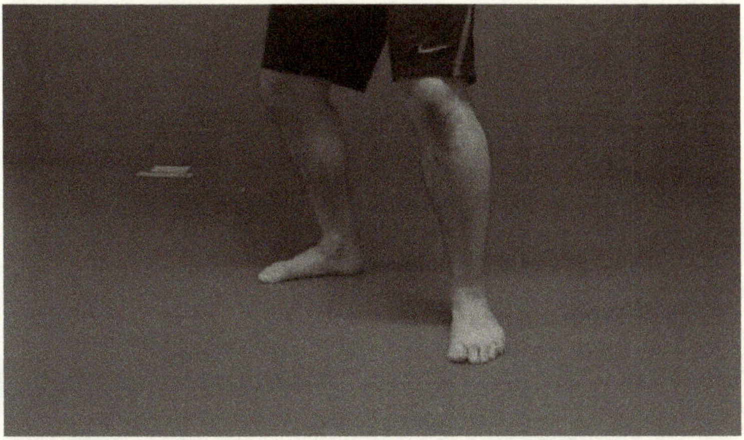

Figure 16: Standing flatfooted means that you have the entire area on the bottom of your feet contacting the ground. This footing is good for establishing a solid base from which to throw punches. In this image, you will see I have the deeper knee bend I spoke of earlier. When throwing punches this knee bend helps me torque my body and throw more power into the punches. We will go over this in more detail further on.

Once you have the stance down, it becomes time to work on movement utilizing this stance. While walking is something people do every day, kickboxing movement is not. The two are fundamentally different, although the result is the same. Not only do the movements differ, but so do the intentions behind the movement. When walking you are only concerned with getting from one place to the next. In kickboxing, you will be concerned with getting from one place to next while avoiding strikes, or other attacks, and setting up strikes or counter strikes. This ability to move while evading or striking is an essential part of kickboxing.

When walking, you place one foot in front of the other to move forward. To move backward, you place one foot behind the other and move backward. When moving forward in a kickboxing stance, you will step forward with your front foot, then slide the back foot forward until you are in your original stance. When moving backward, you will step back with the rear foot then slide the front foot back until you are again in stance. That is the basic idea for movement in stance. The following images will outline movement in detail.

Forward Movement

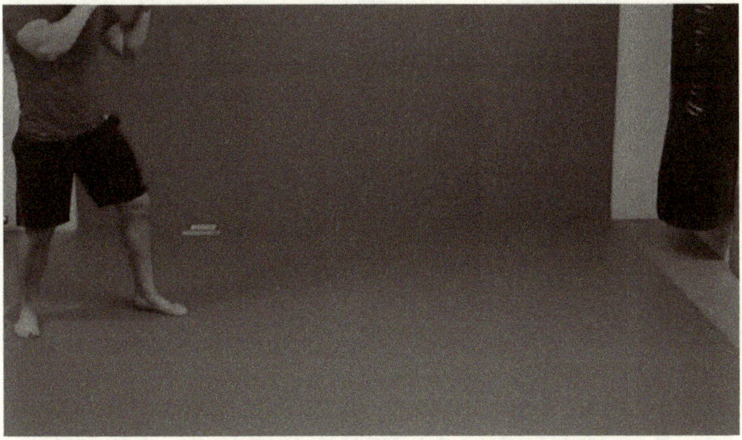

Figure 17: You will be in forward with the stance for movement that I mentioned earlier in figure 2. This is ideal for movement as it allows the feet to flow in a line during movement. This creates smooth footwork and allows you to flow over the ground instead of the traditional walk. This is faster than a walk, but slower than a run. It allows you to maintain your stance. The front foot will slide forward in the direction of the arrow.

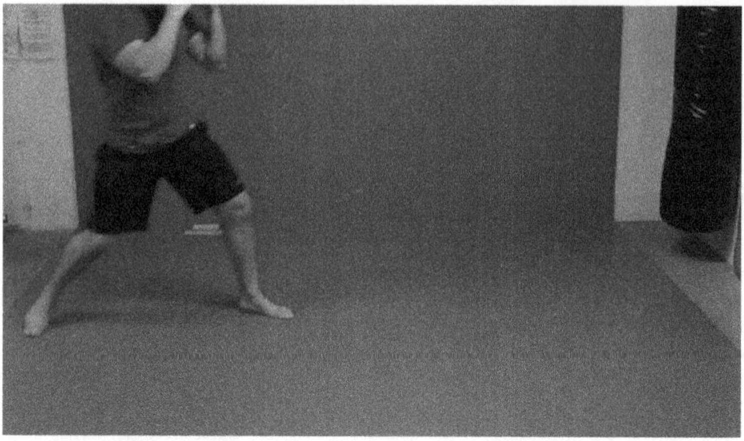

Figure 18: The front foot slides forward. You temporarily have a slightly wider stance from front to back. This is normal and you would not be able to move without some type of increase in stance width. The rear feet will slide forward next.

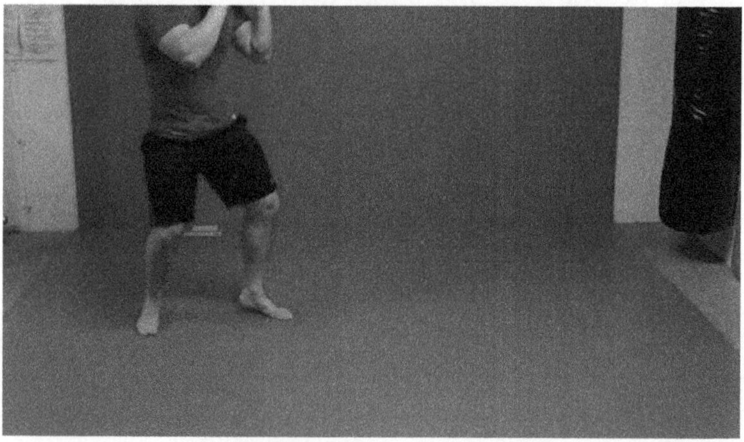

Figure 19: The rear foot slides forward. You have now effectively completed one step. Remember, you are not walking one foot in

front of the other. You are sliding the front foot forward then allowing the rear foot to slide forward behind it. This keeps you in your stance with your lead hand forward. Keep your hands high, head slightly tucked, and move on the balls of your feet. Repeat until you have covered the distance you need to move.

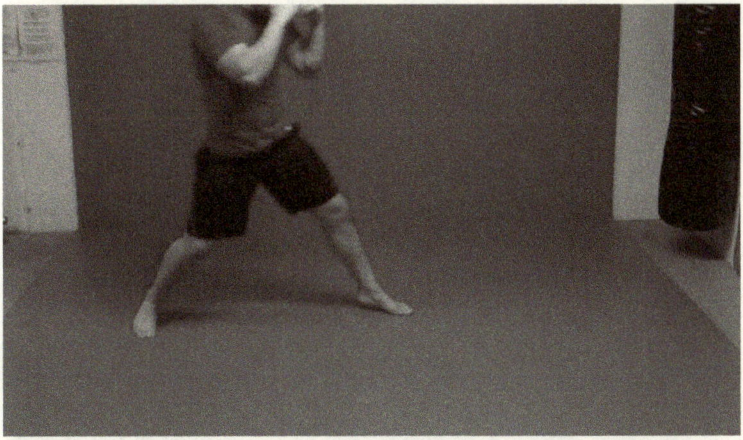

Figure 20: Move forward again. The front foot steps forward first, creating a temporarily larger stance width.

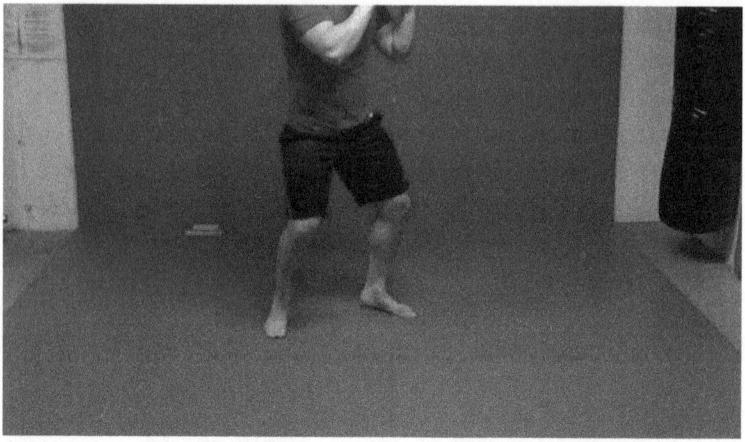

Figure 21: The rear foot then follows and closes the stance. Your lead hand is forward with your hand high and your head slightly tucked. Repeat this until you move the distance you need to achieve.

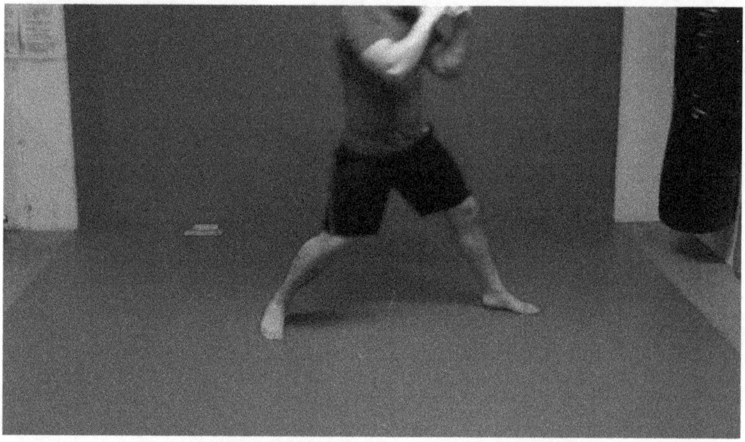

Figure 22: Front foot slides forward.

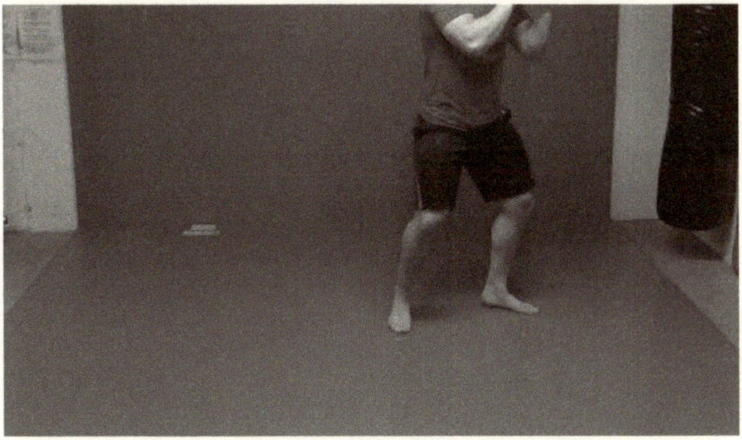

Figure 23: Rear foot slides.

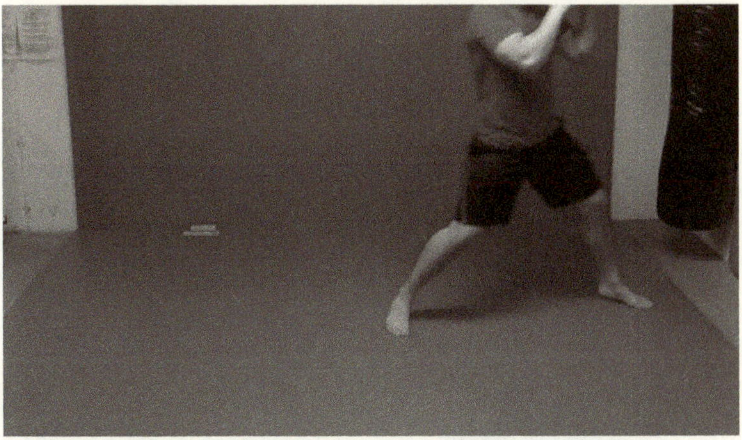

Figure 24: Front foot slides forward.

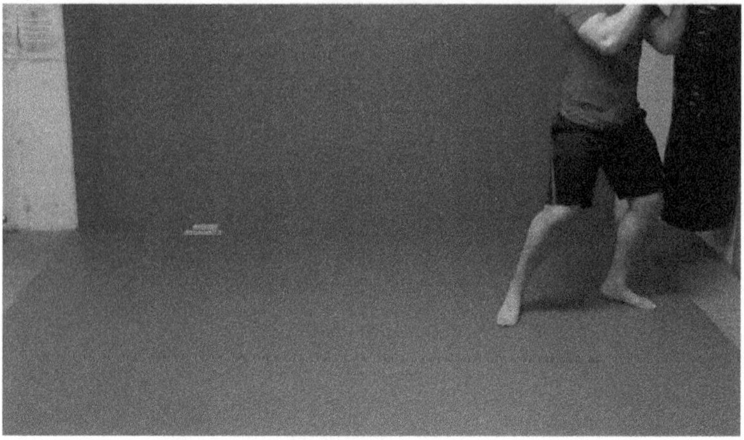

Figure 25: Rear foot slides.

Backward Movement

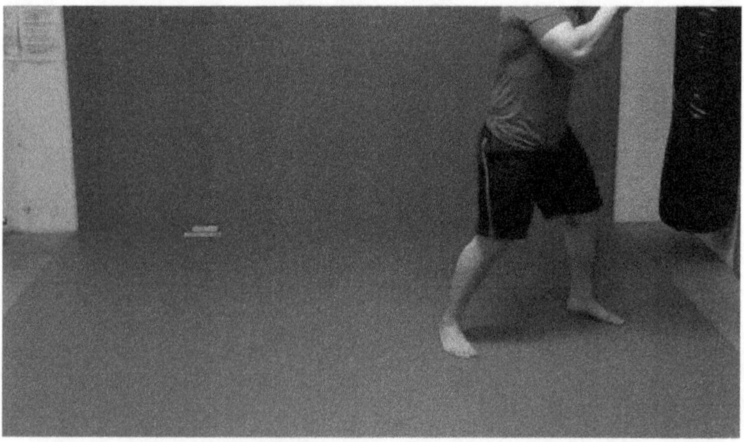

Figure 26: Backward movement is achieved via the same mechanics as forward movement.

The only difference is that you slide with your back foot first.

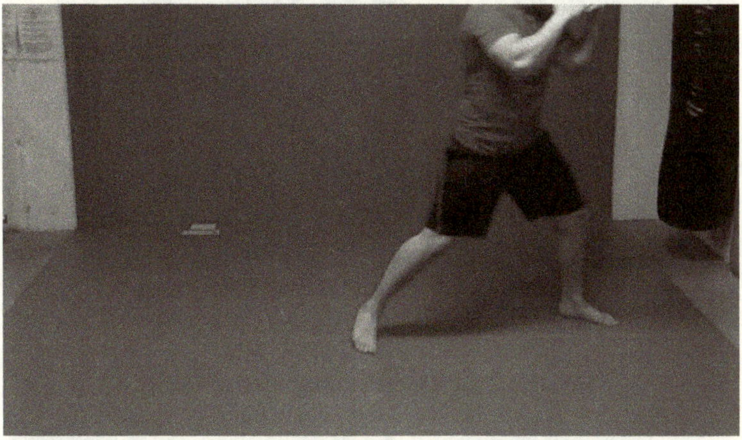

Figure 27: Slide your back foot out while keeping your lead hand forward, hands high, and chin slightly tucked.

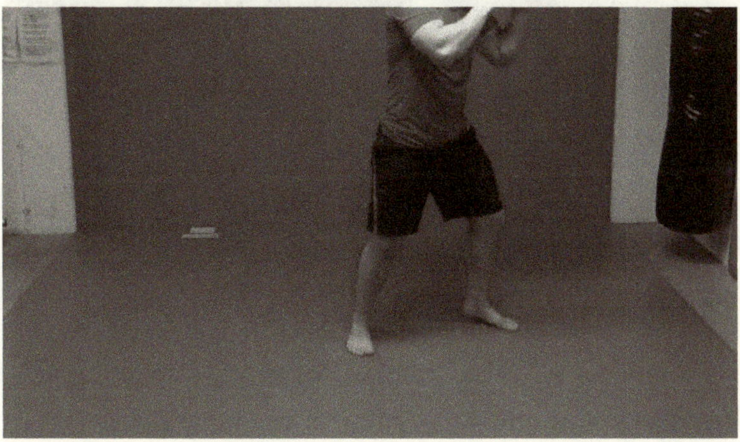

Figure 28: Follow with your front foot.

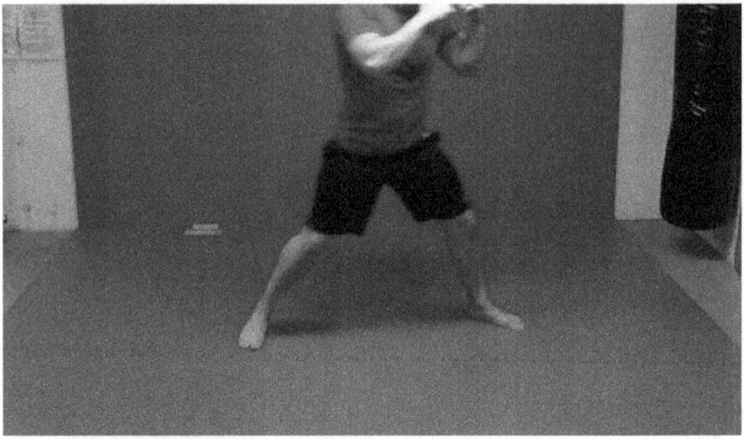

Figure 29: Slide your rear foot.

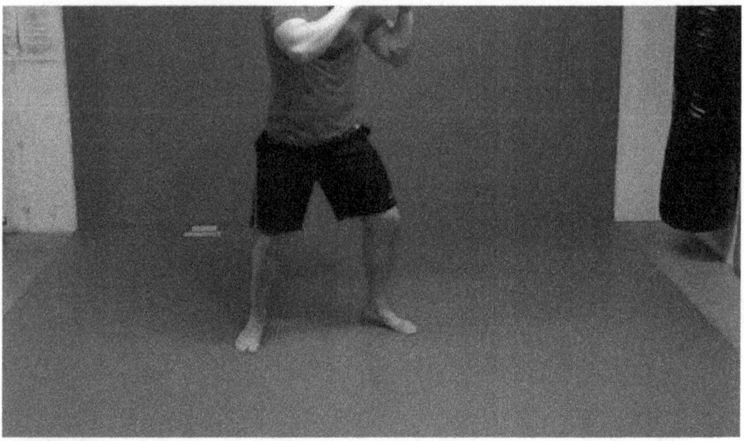

Figure 30: Follow with your front foot.

I realize that this likely sounds boring and tedious. Proper movement is essential to any martial art. Kickboxing is no different. If you take a boxing course, a Tae Kwon Do course, or even a jiu-jitsu course, the fundamentals of standing are going to incorporate proper stance and proper movement.

Do not look at this as a chore. Look at it as a foundation. With improved movement, evasion becomes easier and striking on the go becomes possible. With improved evasion, you take less damage. With increased striking ability, you do more damage. When it comes to kickboxing, or any striking sport, these are necessary abilities. If you don't want to do this, you might as well stop reading now.

I can understand the tediousness of this movement. Practicing moving isn't fun or exciting and it doesn't directly teach how to attack or defend against an opponent. To that end, I suggest incorporating movement work into your warm up and cool down. Every workout should start with a warm up and end with a cool down. I like to do my training sessions in rounds. After my treadmill work, I start with two to three, five-minute warm up rounds on the mat. I practice my footwork and shadow box. This is a great way for you to incorporate footwork (movement). The same can be said of the cool down. Set aside one to two rounds, or a specific time frame, and incorporate some footwork (movement) into it.

Diagonal Movement

Diagonal movement is a bit unique in that it can be done in four directions instead of two, like the front to back movement. Let me illustrate. Imagine that you are standing on the middle of the line in your stance facing the right side of the page. Forward movement would allow you to move to the right side of the page while rear movement would allow you to move to the left side of the page.

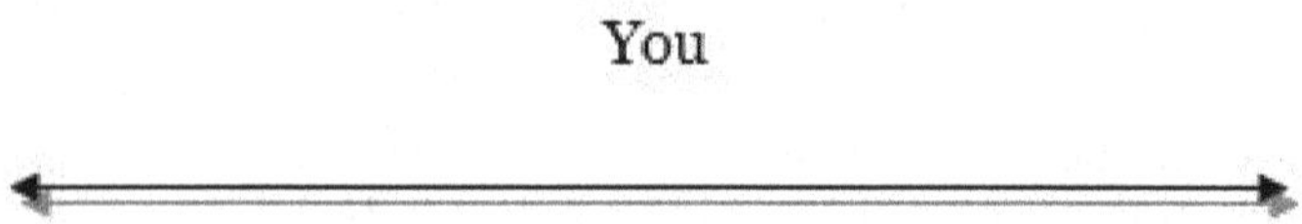

Now, imagine you are in the middle of the circle below and we are looking down at you from top view. The lines represent the diagonal directions you can move. There are four lines with two denoting rear movement and two denoting front movement.

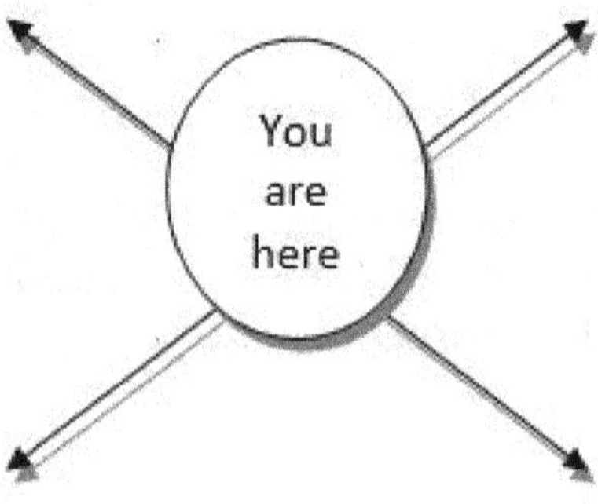

Ideally, diagonal movement does go in four directions, as illustrated by the previous images. However, in order to move forward or backward in one direction, you would need to change stances. This is something we do not want at this point. You should always maintain your stance. Again, let me illustrate, this time with a photo.

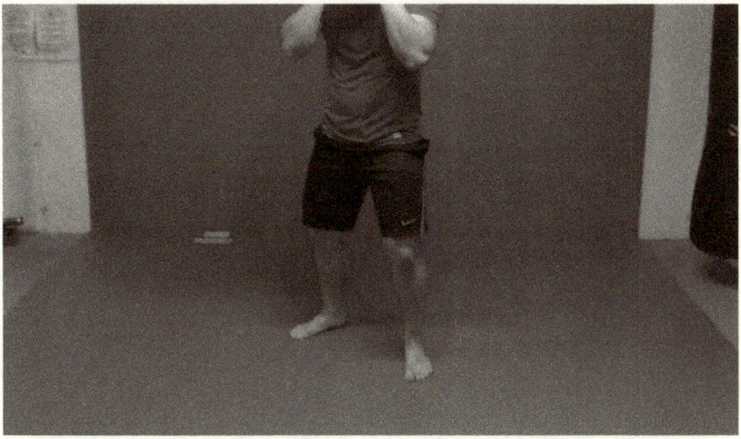

Figure 31: Diagonal movement is done is a forward diagonal or rear diagonal. We will start with rear diagonal movement. Notice the direction indicated by the arrow.

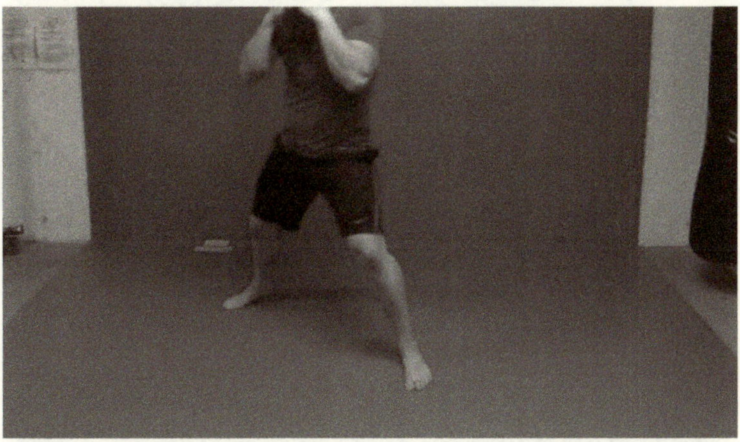

Figure 32: From your normal stance, you step backwards with your rear foot. As with the front to back movement you will be in a larger than normal stance for a moment. Remember to keep your hands high and your stance

facing forward. Keep your eye on your opponent.

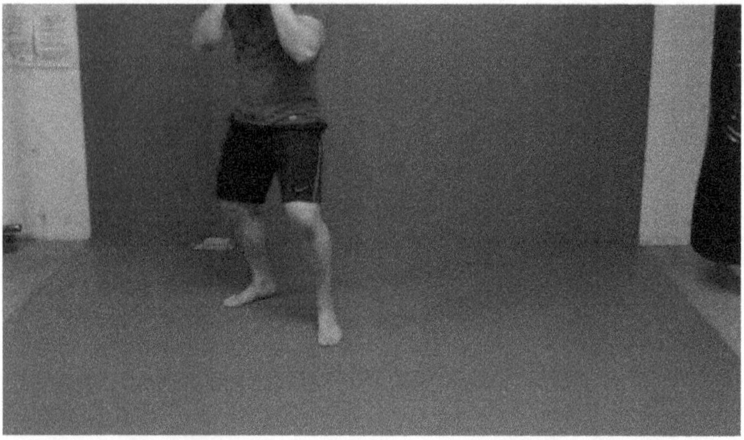

Figure 33: You now slide the front foot back to finish the movement. This is one diagonal step backwards.

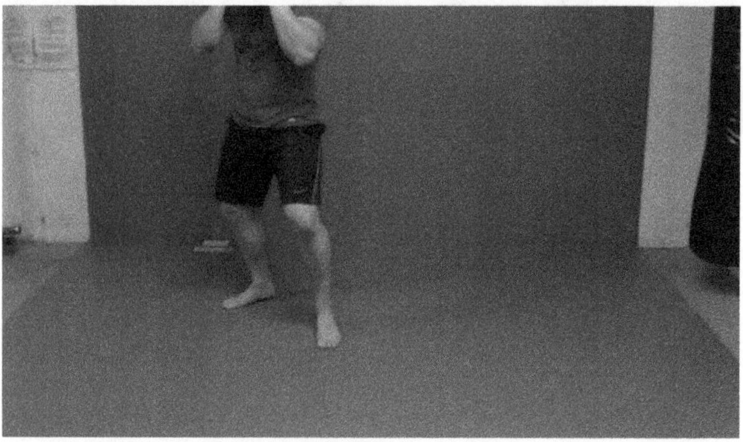

Figure 34: Forward diagonal movement is essentially the same as rear diagonal

movement. The only exception is that you are moving forward.

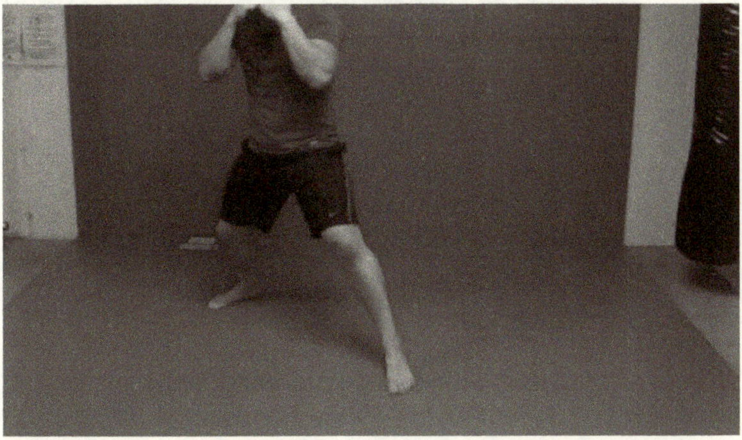

Figure 35: Step forward in a diagonal motion with the front foot. Your hands are high, stance is proper, and your eyes are on your opponent.

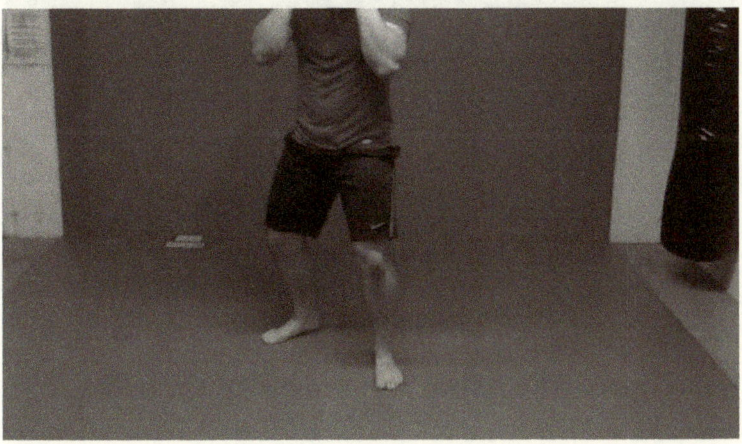

Figure 36: Bring the rear foot forward.

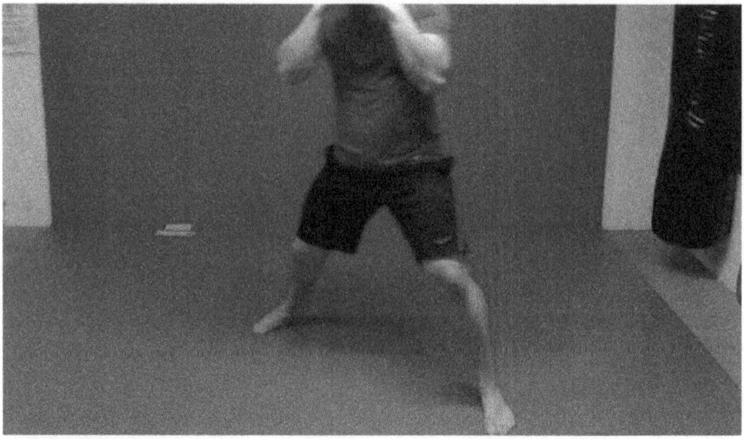

Figure 37: Step forward in a diagonal motion with the front foot. Your hands are high, stance is proper, and your eyes are on your opponent.

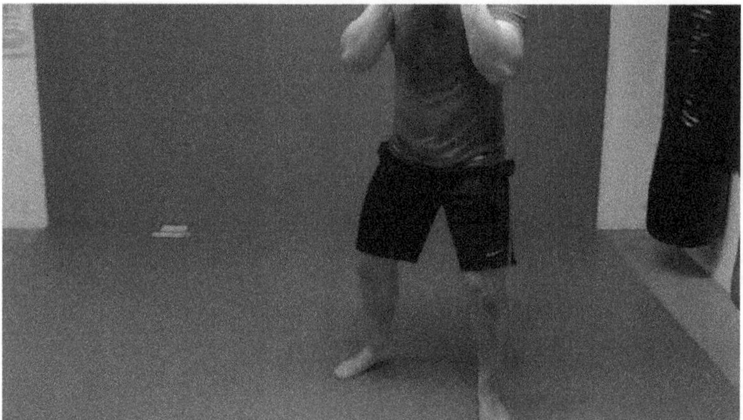

Figure 38: Bring the rear foot forward.

Now, I want to cover one more point with diagonal movement. We have only moved in two directions so far, but, as I mentioned, diagonal movement can technically move in four directions. However, for the time being, I do not want you to move in the other two. If an opponent moves in a manner that would require this time of diagonal movement, you will pivot. The reason for this is that the other diagonal movement causes you to either step forward with you rear leg or step backward with you front leg without moving the other leg first. This causes a change in stance. For now, you want to maintain your stance. Let me show you what I mean.

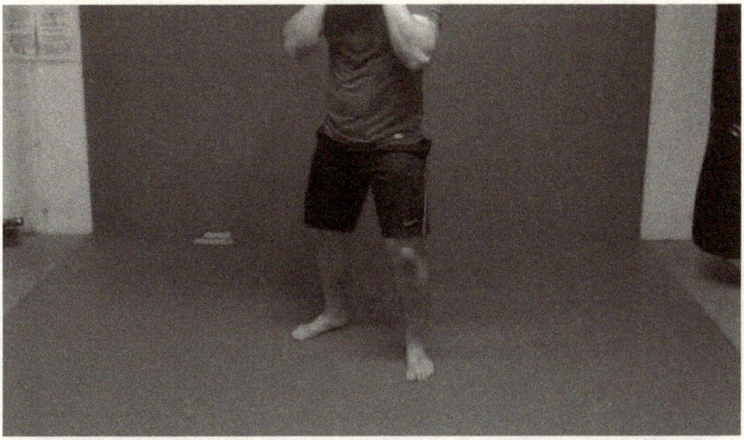

Figure 39: In order to move diagonally you would need to step forward with your back foot. This would cause you to change stance. In this case, the change is from an orthodox stance to a southpaw stance. While it might seem a simple change, standing in a different stance can be awkward until you get used to it. That takes practice. For now, pivot or side step if someone moves in a manner that would result in this type of diagonal movement from you.

Side to Side Movement

Side-to-side movemnt is performed just as it sounds. Using one leg, you step to the side you wish to move and immediately follow with the opposite leg. For a moment, your stance will be slightly wider and you will in a more forward stance. Once you bring the second leg across to finish the side step, your stance will again be normal. Allow me to illustrate.

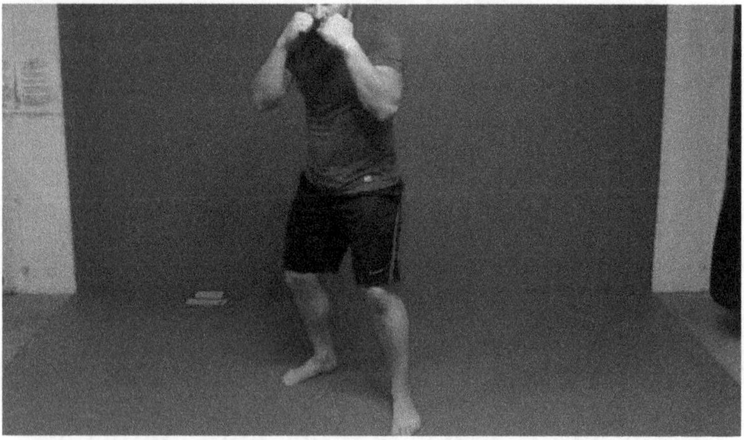

Figure 40: This is your normal stance. It is staggered with your lead leg forward and your rear leg back. From here, you will initiate the side step with one leg or the other.

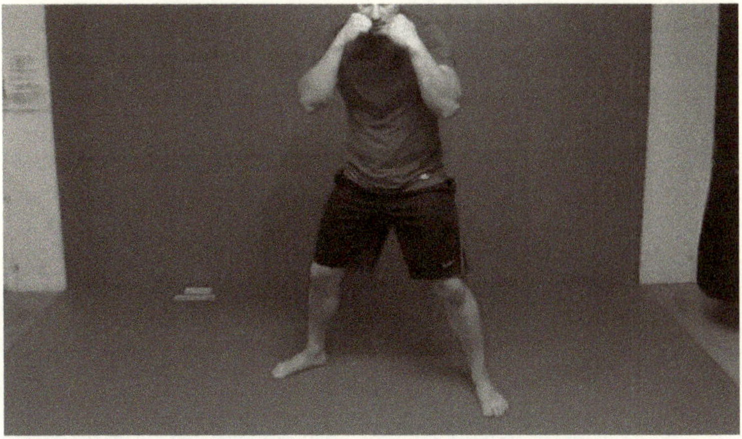

Figure 41: In this image, I side step with my lead leg by moving it to the outside of my body. This is how the side step should always start in this manner. There should be no crossing of the legs.

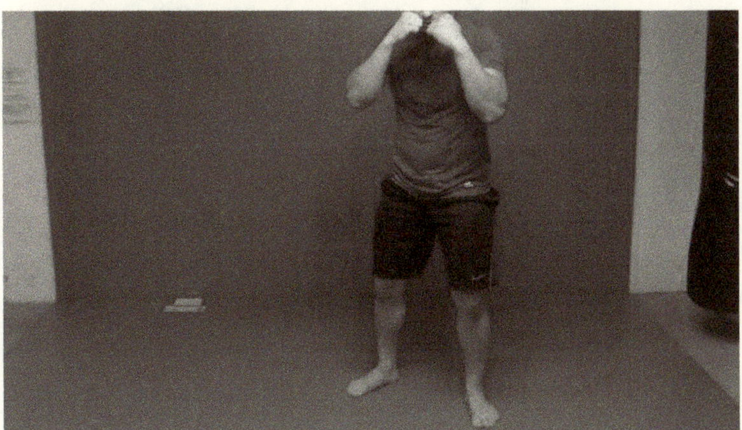

Figure 42: I now follow my front leg with my rear leg. This closes the wider than normal stance and put me back in my original stance.

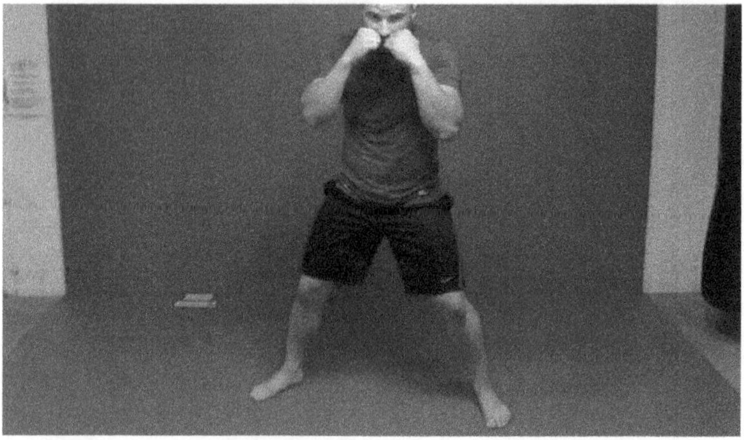

Figure 43: I now step to the right by moving my back leg in the direction that I want to move.

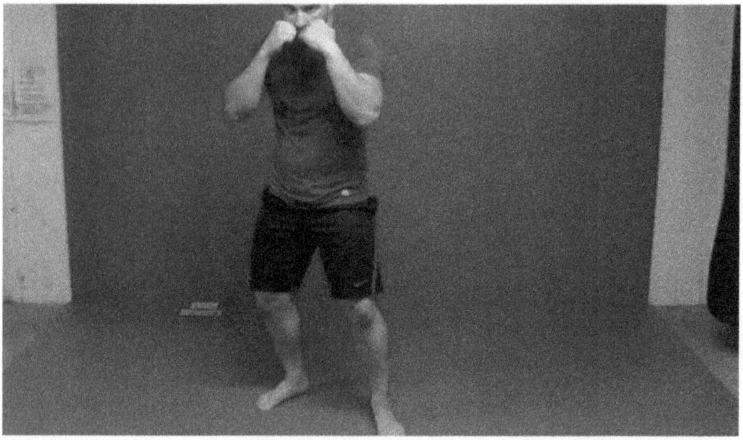

Figure 44: I follow my rear leg with my front leg. I have now completed the side step.

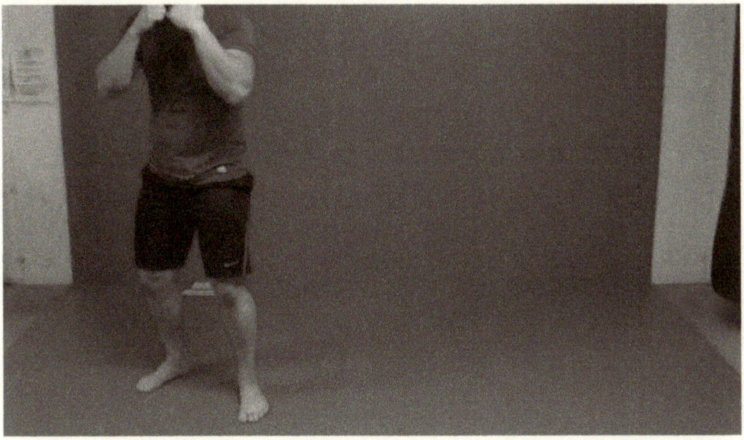

Figure 45: The motion for the side step is the same regardless of how many times it is done. Always start the side step with the leg closest to the direction you want to move...

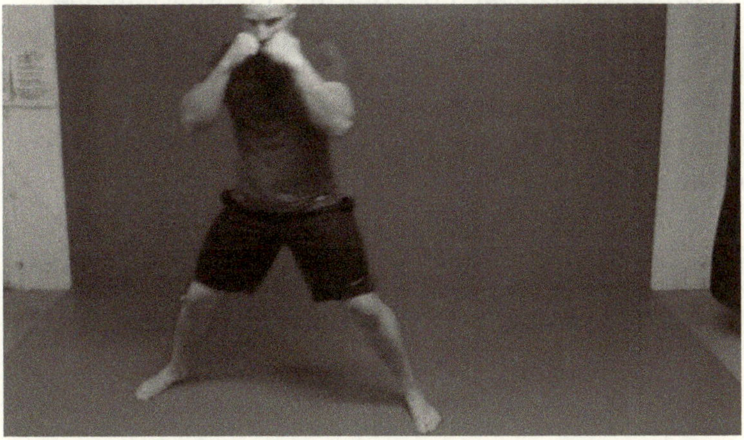

Figure 46: step with that leg first...

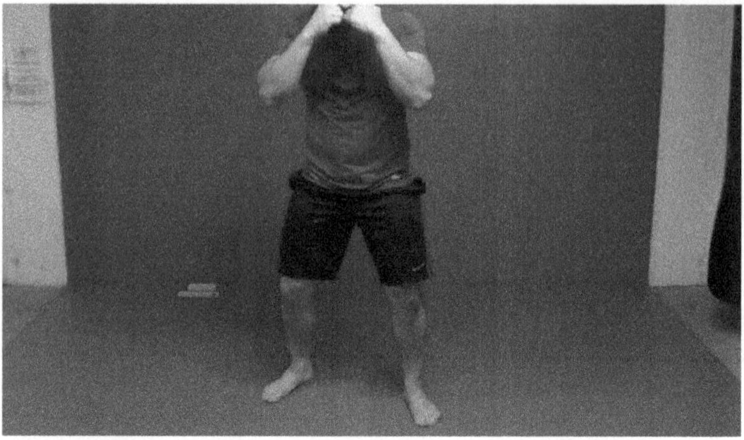

Figure 47: then follow with the other leg.

Pivoting

Pivoting is performed by rotating (pivoting) on one foot. This pivot can occur on the front or the rear foot, although it generally occurs on the front foot. The next series of photos will outline how to pivot on the front foot. Pivoting on the rear foot is essentially the same.

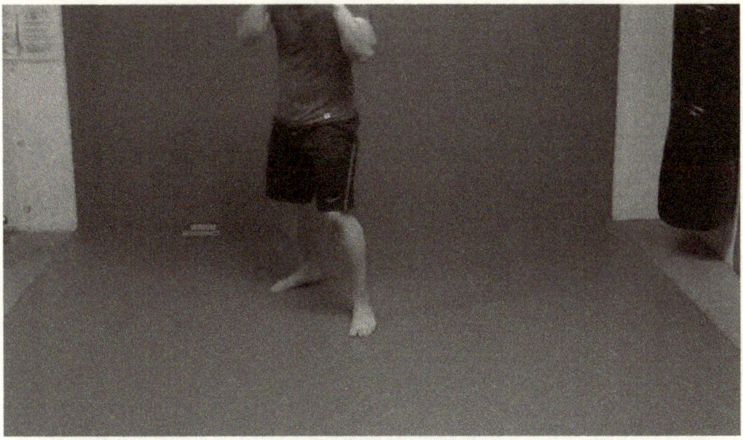

Figure 48: In this image, I am standing in an orthodox stance. Position yourself in the same way. You are going to pivot to face your right side. This will cause your rear foot to pivot toward your left side.

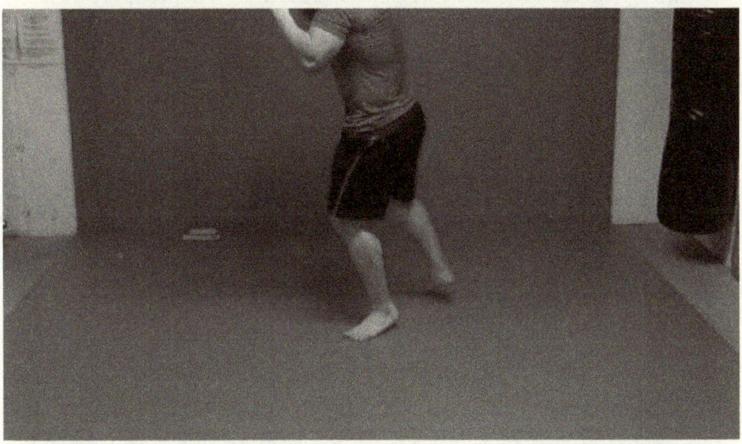

Figure 49: This image shows me in mid-pivot. Notice my rear foot is slightly off the ground as it is the foot moving. I am balancing on the ball of my front foot to facilitate the pivot. If

you stand flat-footed, the pivot is difficult and you could tweak (sprain) your ankle.

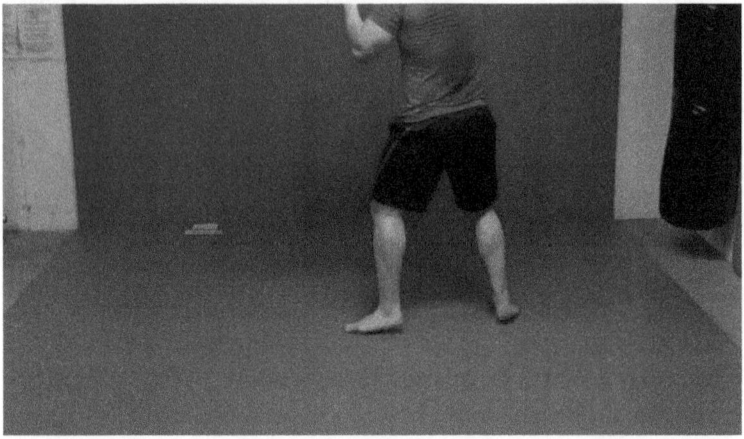

Figure 50: I have completed the pivot. Notice that I am still on the balls of my feet (it is a bit exaggerated for effect). This is to facilitate continued movement. If I wanted to throw punches, I would seat back on my feet for a flat-footed power stance.

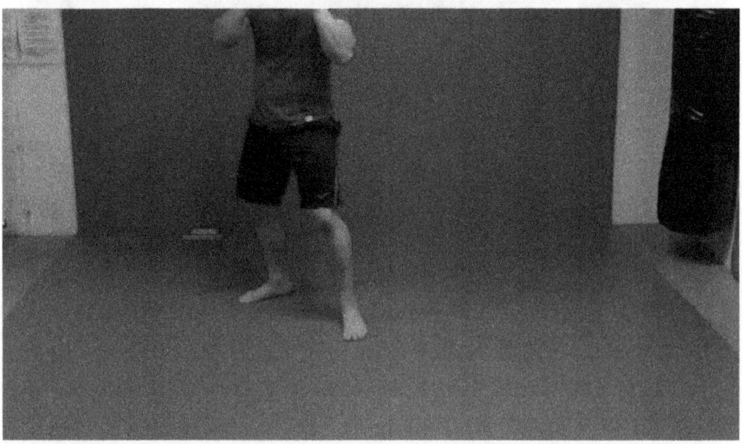

Figure 51: Now I will show you how to pivot to the other direction. You will start from the original stance. Notice in the image I am again in my standard stance facing forward. From here, I will pivot (rotate) to face my left side. My rear foot will pivot to my right.

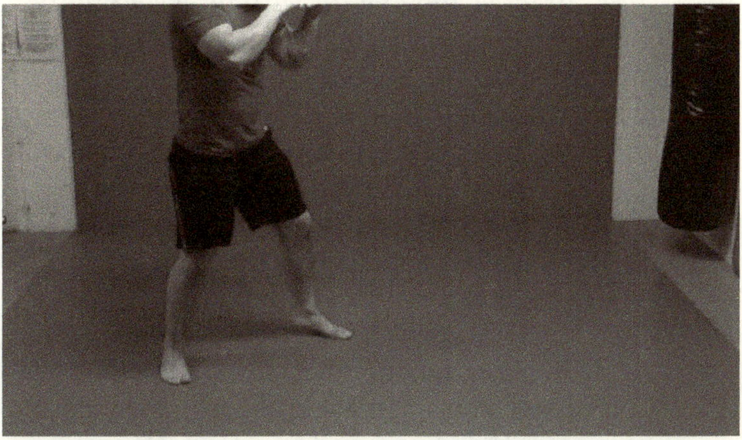

Figure 52: You pivot in the same manner as the first pivot. It is that simple. Pivoting is an easy move to perform but it can take practice to become fluid with it.

Chapter Review

In this chapter, we have reviewed how you should stand (stance) and how you should move (movement) when practicing kickboxing. Understanding these principles are essential to kickboxing. You should have a working knowledge of them as you proceed forward.

Practice Suggestions

- Practice each set of movements individually first. Practice moving forward for a set number of repetitions or for time before moving to the next movement.
- Use a predetermined rep range or time frame. 5, 10, 15, or 20 steps in one direction is a good place to start. For example, do ten forward steps in one direction, pivot, then do ten steps forward again. If you prefer time, try using intervals of 15 seconds such as 15, 30, 45, etc.
- Once you are comfortable with movement in one direction, move in two directions, then three, and so on. For example, step forward ten steps and then backward ten steps. Once you are comfortable with that, add in ten side steps in each direction.

Chapter 2: Defense – Blocking Punches and Evasion

Defense is essential to surviving a fight. While being able to attack will incapacitate an opponent, proper defense will keep you from being incapacitated. Imagine for second a man running into a fight with his hands down and trying to swing punches from the waist. This man is leaving his head wide open for a punch and runs the risk of being knocked out.

Now let's imagine his opponent. This man has his hands high and easily blocks the telegraphed punches thrown from the first man's waist. The second man in turn capitalizes on the first man's exposed head and punches him in the face, knocking him out. This is a very real scenario and one you want to avoid.

Defense encompasses blocking and evasion. Both aspects are equally important. Blocking allows you to defend against a strike and prevent it from doing damage to important tissue, such as allowing a hook to hit the arm instead of the head. Evasion prevents the punch from ever landing and this is the ideal scenario.

The Rock Back

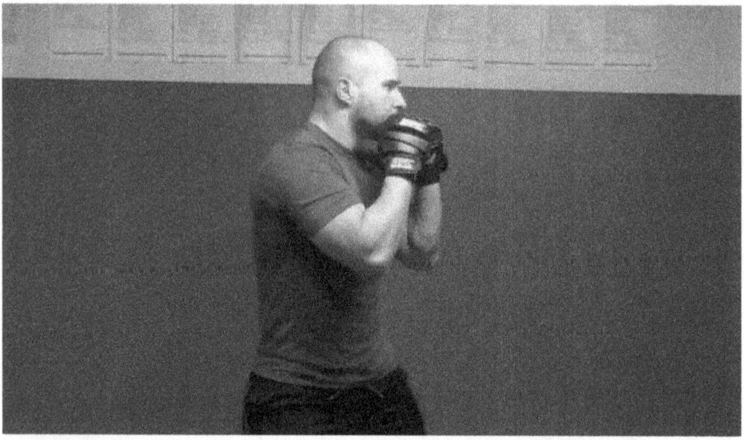

Figure 53: The rock back is my favorite evasive maneuver. It allows me to stay in the pocket and not get hit. It can be used to avoid any type of head punch. The best part about it is that it is simple to learn and perform. The rock back simple requires that you lean back. To perform the move, you start in your normal stance.

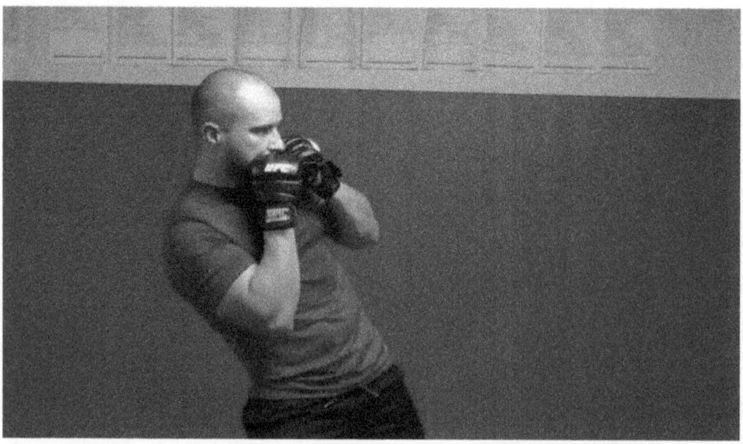

Figure 54: You then just lean back at the waist. Be sure to keep your hands high. Unless your opponent is right on top of you, their punch will miss in this position. Remember, like all moves, this has to be applied with proper timing. If it is not, you likely will get punched in the face.

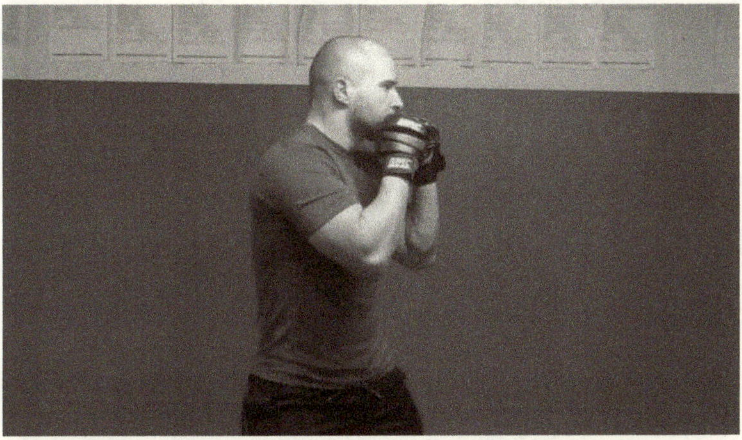

Figure 55: Return to the start position. Remember to always keep your hands high to protect your face.

Slipping

Slipping is one of the best-known evasive maneuvers in boxing. It is used to avoid straight punches, the jab, and the cross. Slipping is performed by moving your body to the outside of the attacker's punching arm as the punch is thrown. Like all moves, this must be applied with proper timing to be effective. This is effective for boxing environments as well as kickboxing or MMA environments. The following images will illustrate. This is my second favorite evasive maneuver.

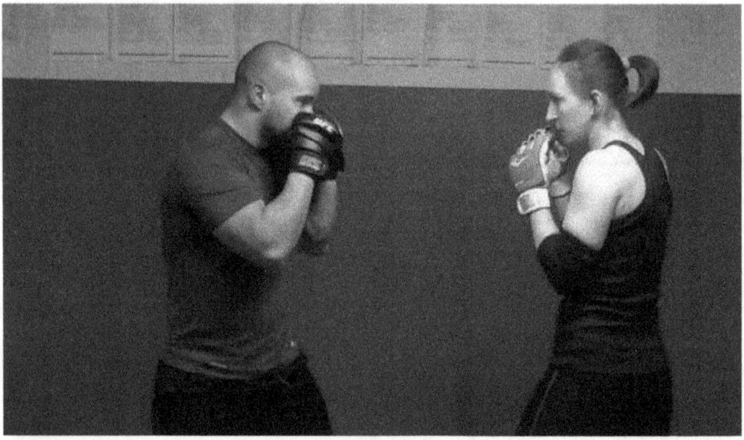

Figure 56: In this image, my partner and I are squared up. We are "in the pocket" and ready to bang (not really but for illustrative purposes). From this position, the slip is performed to avoid a punch.

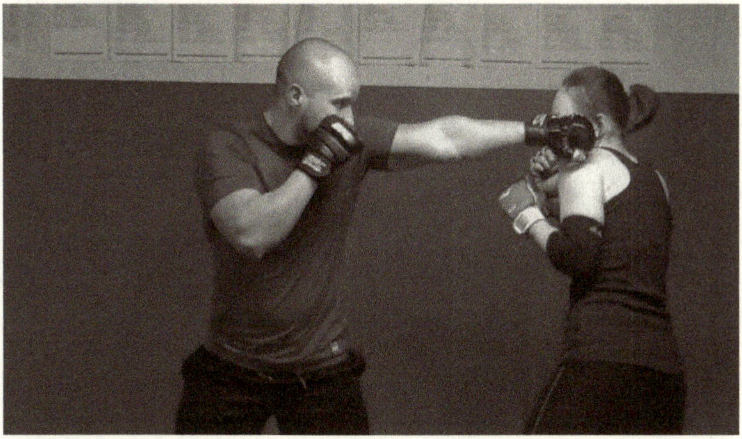

Figure 57: I throw a jab toward my partner. She leans to the side slightly to avoid the punch. Notice that she is NOT doing a dramatic lean to the side. There is no need for this. You should move only the minimal amount needed to avoid the punch. This allows you to react quickly and efficiently. The less distance you move, the quicker you can return to the start position. A good rule of thumbs is to move six to eight inches to the side.

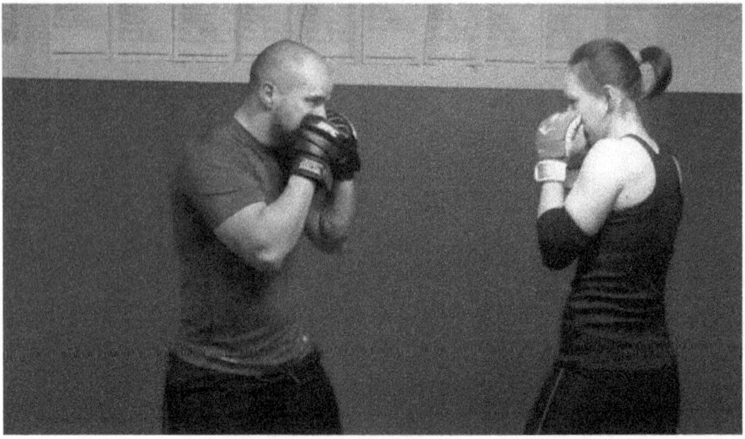

Figure 58: Return to start position.

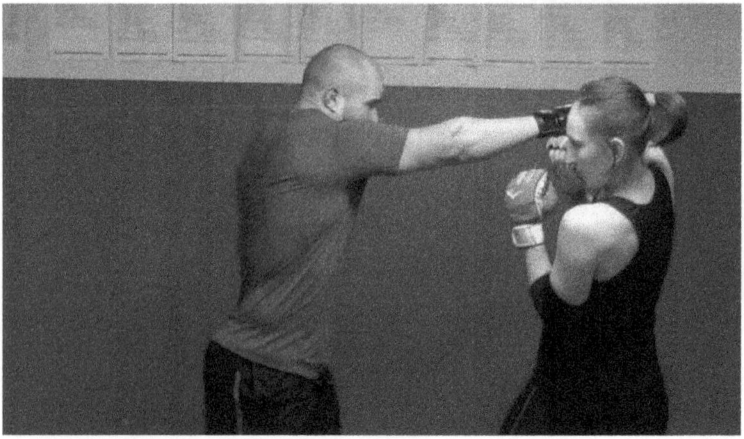

Figure 59: I now throw the cross. My partner leans to the outside of the punch. Remember, always move to the outside of the punch. If you slip to the inside, you could move into a second punch.

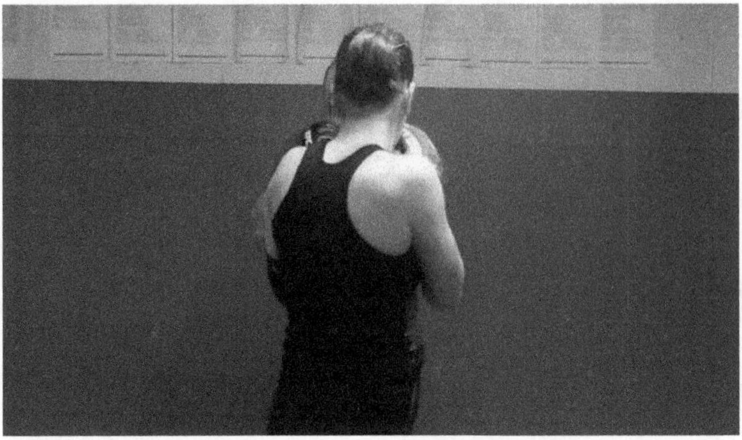

Figure 60: Return to start position.

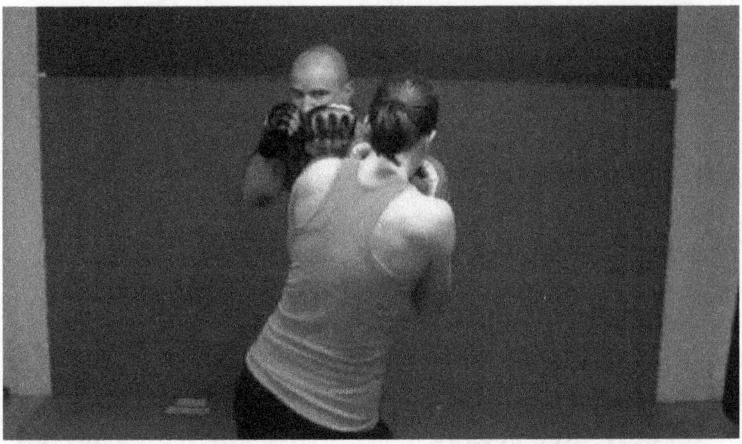

Figure 61: Here is a rear view of my partner slipping the jab. Notice that she has not done some dramatic lean, but rather moved roughly six to eight inches to the outside of the punch. This has allowed her to avoid the punch.

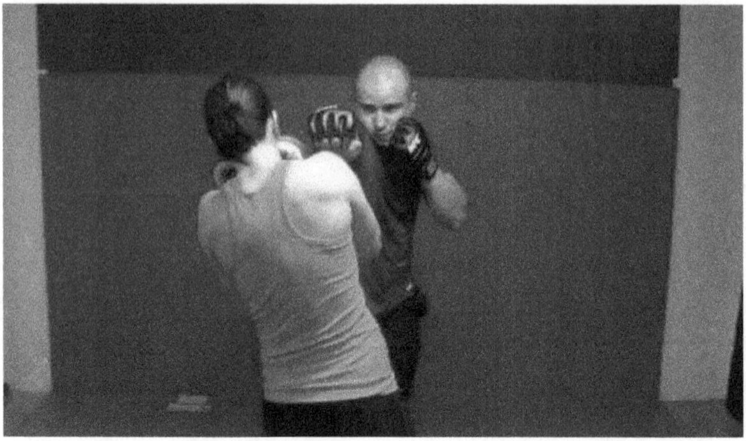

Figure 62: My partner does the same thing here with the cross. In both of these images, she has plenty of space between her and the punch. She could have slipped even less, especially with the cross but this is effective.

Bob-N-Weave

The Bob-N-Weave is a boxing staple. It is not as common in kickboxing or MMA due to the potential for knee strike. In kickboxing, a person performing the Bob-N-Weave leaves themselves open to a knee to the face at the bottom of the movement. However, in a boxing oriented setting this move is efficient. I am not a big fan of the move due to the timing required to effectively perform it and the potential for a knee strike. The rock back is a much better alternative. When possible, use the rock back move instead of the Bob-N-Weave. However, there are many people who use this move with success, so it is essential to learn.

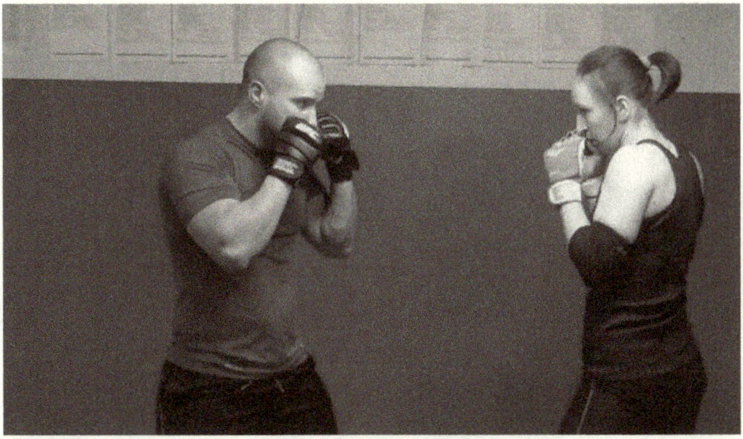

Figure 63: The Bob-N-Weave starts in the basic stance. In this image, I am again the attacker and my partner is the defender. The move is used to evade a hook shot.

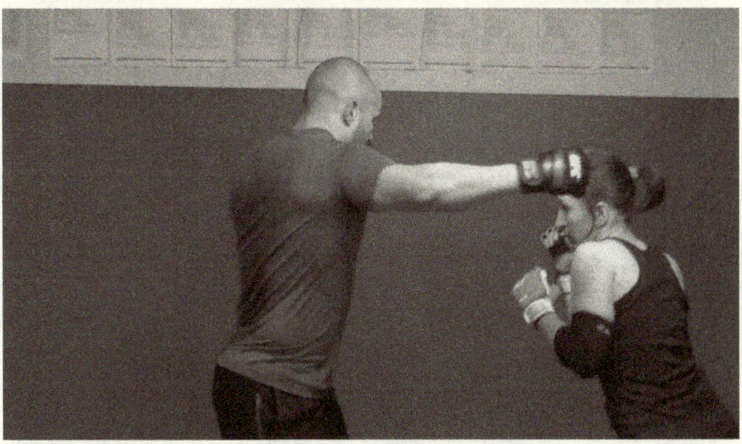

Figure 64: I throw a right hook. The defender ducks under the hook in a "U" shaped manner moving from right to left. In this image, she

has begun her descent as my punch is approaching her.

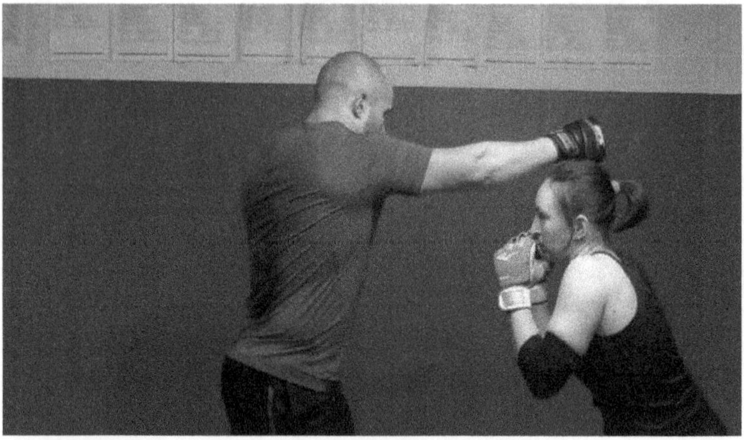

Figure 65: The defender continues her "U" motion, which causes her to travel under my punch as it moves. Again, she is moving right to left since my punch is moving toward her left side. Notice that the punch is just above her head. This is fine. The "U" does not have to be excessive.

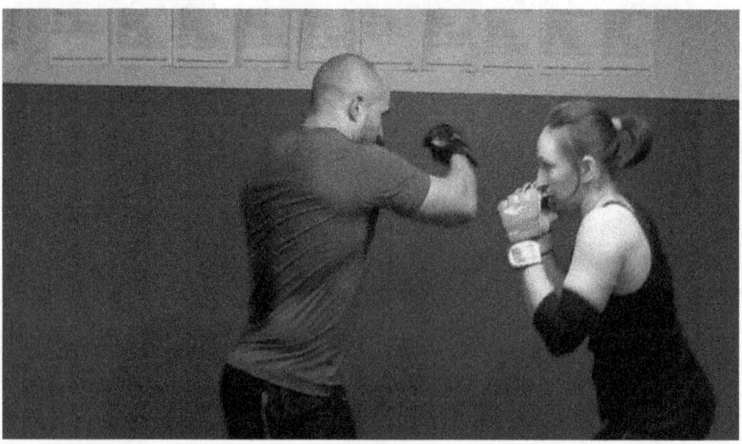

Figure 66: The defender is now on the ascent part of the "U". My punch has now cleared her head and she is moving back to the start position.

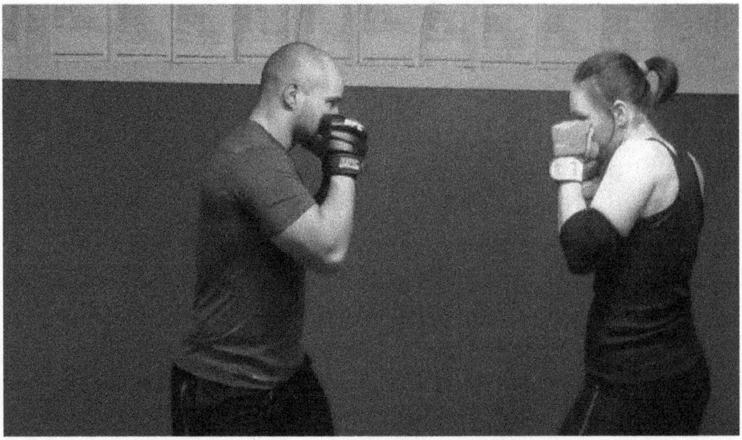

Figure 67: The defender has returned to start position, as have I.

Head Movement (and Movement in General)

Head movement may be one of the most underrated defensive maneuvers. It is effective at avoiding punches, but also at disrupting an attacker's throwing pattern. A still target is easier to aim for, while a moving target means the striker has to move with the target to hit it. This can be enough to stifle an attacker's offense.

Head movement can also allow you to set up strikes and counter strikes easier. When throwing strikes there is always some kind of "tel" or form of telegraphing. Telegraphing is a movement before the strike is thrown. With punches, it is the movement of the shoulder before the punch is thrown. For a round kick, it is the turn of the hip before the kick is thrown.

When a person utilizes movement, in this case head movement, the tel is harder to see. This is because you are already in movement so, the attacking movement can be mistaken for general movement instead of striking movement. Some of the best strikers use head movement, or other types of movements such as feints, to confuse their opponent.

Head movement, and movement in general, is not confined to boxing, kickboxing of any one martial art, or form of combat. It is not even confined to stand up fighting. Ground fighting methods can benefit from movement as well. Again, let's look at the example of the still target vs. the moving target. If you are laying on the ground with a person in your **guard** (this is a jiu-jitsu term if you want to reference it) and a person is trying to hit you, you don't just want to lay there. You want to move either by **shrimping** (another jiu-jitsu term), obtaining wrist/arm control, or using some other defensive movement.

Movement is something I cannot stress enough. It is an essential part of defense and can keep you from getting hurt. Utilize movement as often as possible and look to perfect movements that work for you. Protect yourself, my friend.

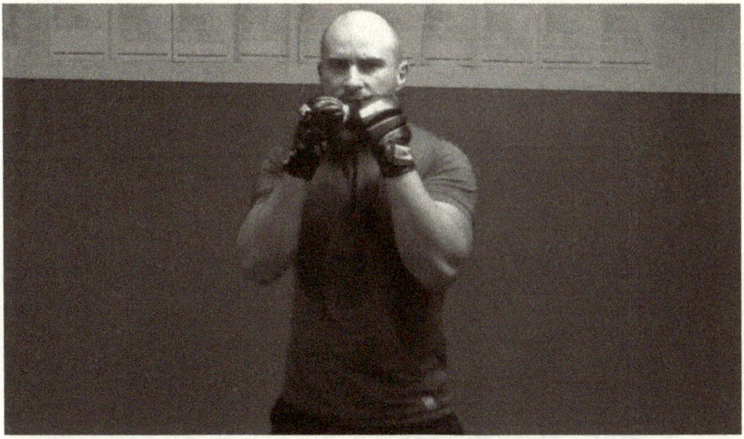

Figure 68: Head movement is easy to perform, but it can be hard to implement in a fight. Head movement simply means moving the head and it starts from the basic stance (although it can be used in any position, see the previous paragraph). Head movement is actually a misleading term. The "head" movement actually occurs at the waist. You lean, bend, or twist at the waist to move the head from harm's way.

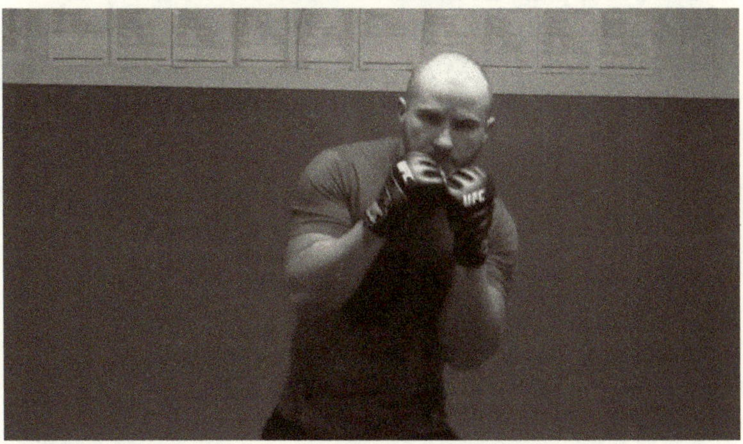

Figure 69: In this image, I have moved to the side. Essentially, I am slipping (see the slipping section). This movement can be used to confuse the opponent and make them throw a punch in the wrong direction.

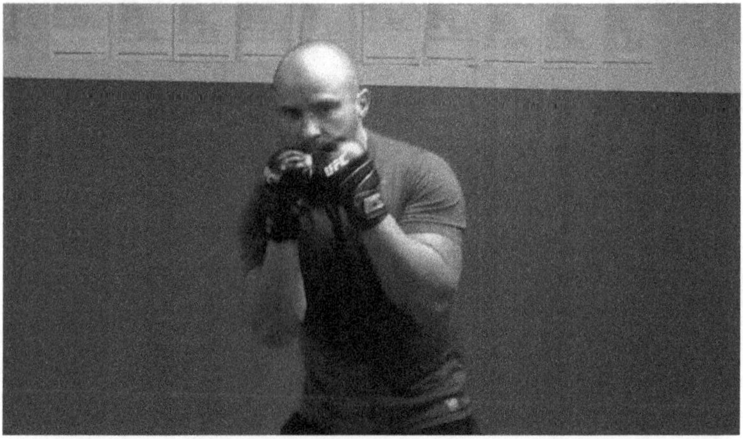

Figure 70: Now I am leaning to the opposite side as if slipping. Again, this can be used to confuse the opponent. Conversely, I can also throw a punch from here. Potentially, my opponent thinks I am just moving for evasive purposes. If I throw an uppercut to the head or a hook the body, I might catch my opponent off guard.

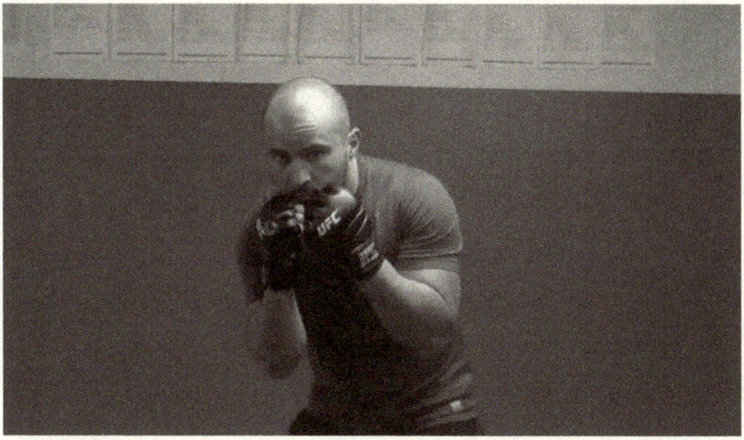

Figure 71: In this image, I am ducking down as if to do the Bob-N-Weave. While the Bob-N-Weave is used to avoid hook punches, it can also be used as part of general head movement to confuse an opponent and avoid strikes. At any point in the movement, I can throw a punch should the opportunity arise. For this half-ducked position, I can throw a hook to the body or explode upwards to deliver a hook to an exposed jaw.

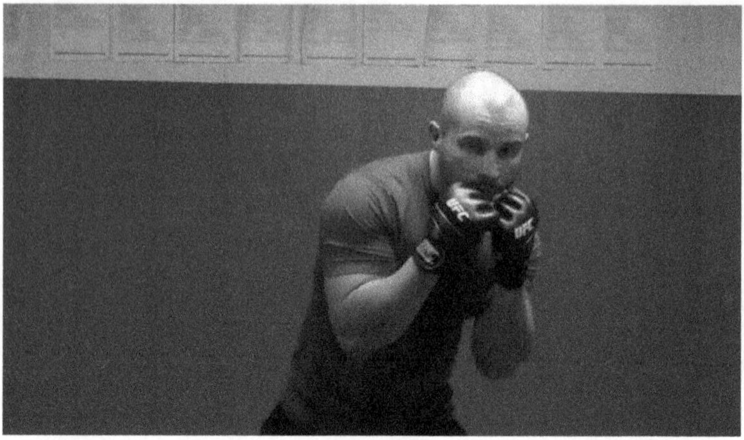

Figure 72: The same idea applies here. I am coming back up from the Bob-N-Weave. From here, I can throw a hook or a straight shot with my left hand. My body is already torqued in that direction and ready to spring. Keep this is mind as you practice head movement and try to incorporate strikes.

Chapter Review

In this chapter, we have reviewed how you avoid and defend against punches. Properly blocking punches, or avoiding them altogether prevents you from taking damage. This can make the difference between winning and losing a fight. Practice the included movements until they become second nature.

Practice Suggestions

- Practice each of the movements in the chapter until you have a feel for them.
- Practice with a partner whenever possible to make the movements more realistic.
- Try the movements in different orders to avoid getting stuck in a pattern and to help the moves become second nature.

Chapter 3: Attacking with Punches

Punching is striking at its most basic. Every person has, at one point or another, thrown a punch, whether in anger or in jest. At a glance, throwing a punch is a simple task. You just have to push your arm out. However, this does not make for a good punch. A proper punch follows a prescribed technique that maximizes form and speed to translate into power. That is what we will cover in this chapter.

There are only several different punches in striking: Jab, cross, front hook, rear hook, front uppercut, and rear uppercut. These are all the basic punches and other punches, such as the body shot, are just variations of these. Take notice that I referred to "front" and "rear" punches as opposed to left or right. I use this terminology because it is a universal language for both the orthodox and the southpaw stances. If you tell an orthodox person to throw a left, it will be a front shot. If you tell a southpaw person to throw a left, if will be a rear shot.

I say other punches are variations of these punches because, in essence, they are. A hook to the body is simply a variation of the hook. A jab to the body is a variation of the jab. It is that simple. The same idea applies to punches from the clinch, on the ground, and everything in between.

The Jab

The jab is the most basic punch in kickboxing and boxing. It is thrown off the lead hand. Notice that I say the lead hand and not the right or left hand. A person who stands in an orthodox position will have their left hand as their lead hand, while the Southpaw person will have their right hand as their lead hand. Due to this, I refer to the lead (front) and rear hands. That way the idea applies to both Orthodox and Southpaw stances.

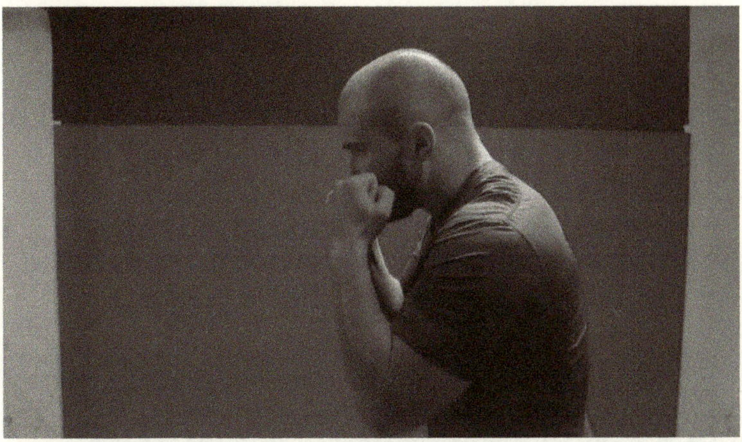

Figure 73: This is the starting position for the jab.

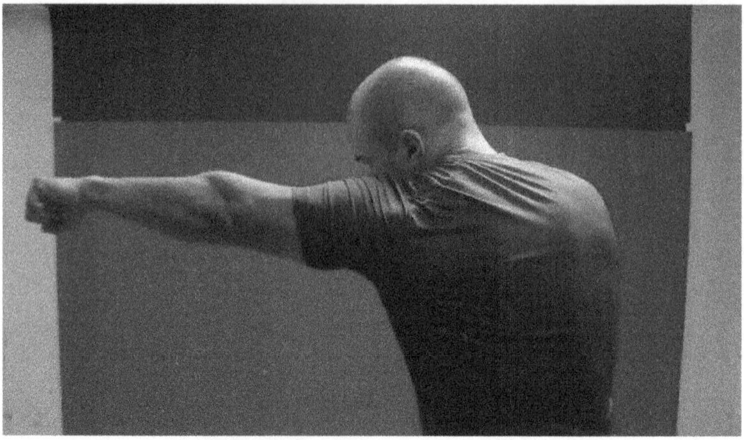

Figure 74: Throw the jab straight out from the body. The punch is thrown quickly with a complete turnover of the hand. Notice how the back of my hand is facing skyward. My fist is closed and my knuckles are forward. The elbow should stay tight and not flair out excessively when this punch is thrown. If the elbow is flaring out, then correct it.

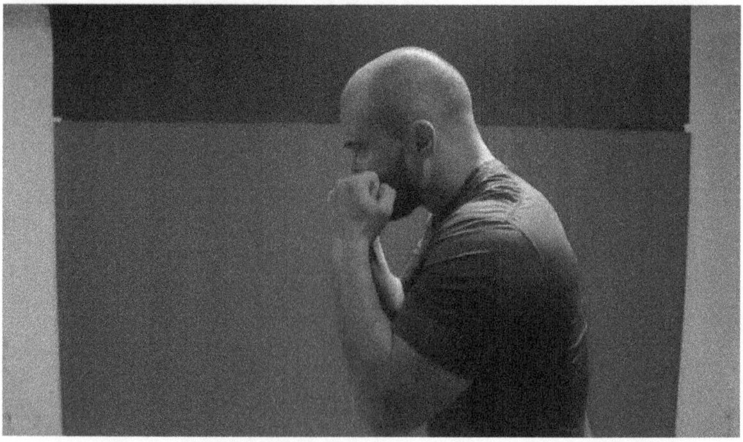

Figure 75: Return the punch to the start position. This should be a quick return. Do not leave your hand "hanging" in the air or allow it to return slowly. This exposes your face and leaves you vulnerable to a counter strike. Ideally, the punch should return as quickly as it was extended.

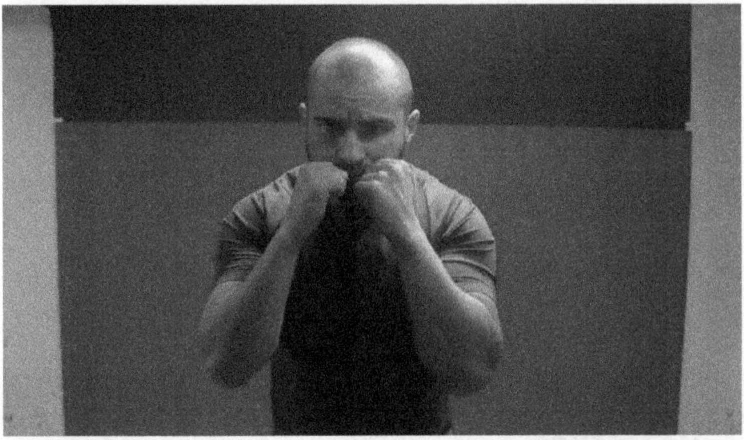

Figure 76: This is the front view of the jab.

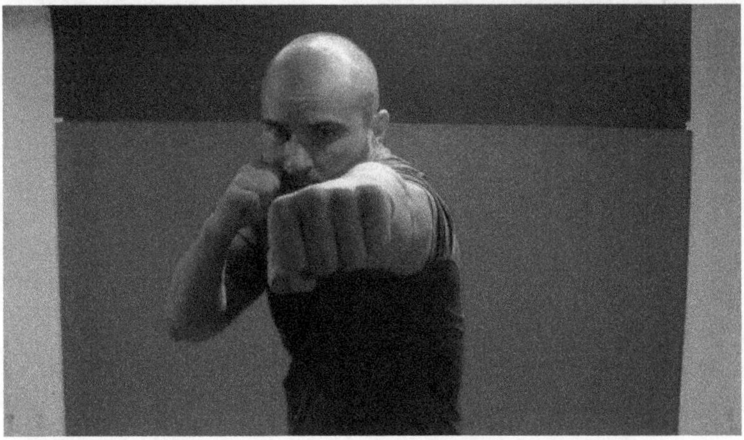

Figure 77: Throw the punch.

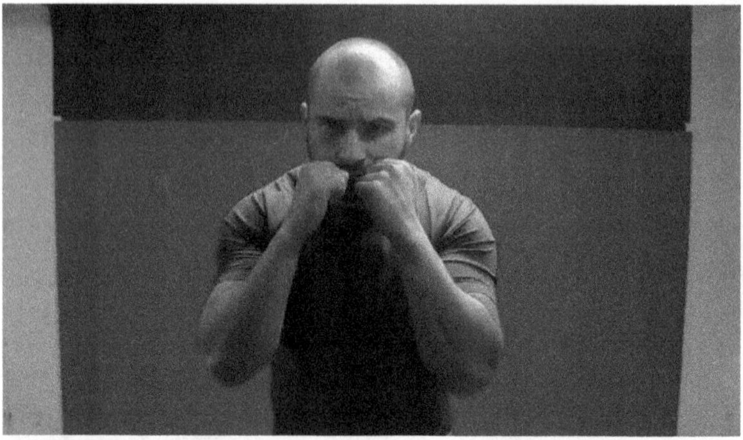

Figure 78: Return to the start position.

The Cross

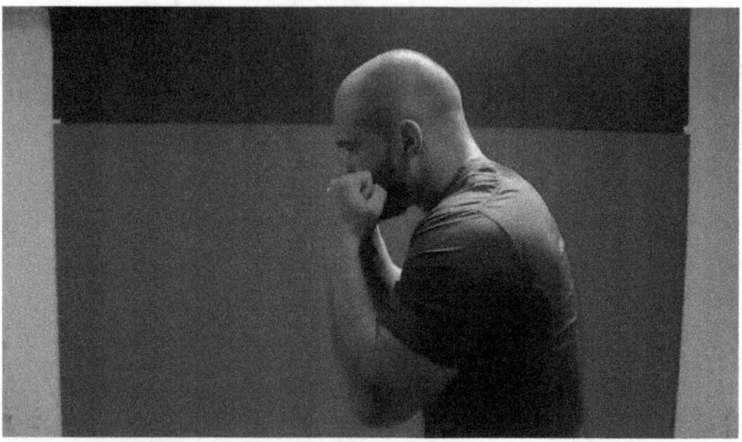

Figure 79: The jab is thrown in the same manner as the jab except with the rear hand. You will throw the punch straight out in a quick manner and return it just as quick.

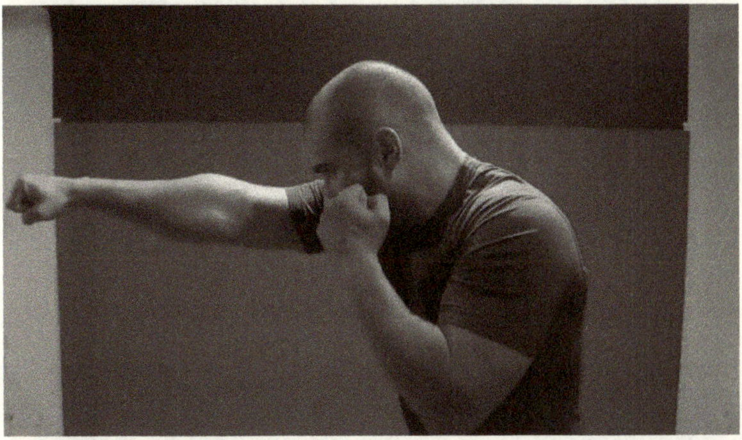

Figure 80: Notice how my non-punching hand is protecting my face. Whenever you throw a punch with one hand, the other hand should be protecting the face. Notice how my punching had is completely turned over and my knuckles are forward.

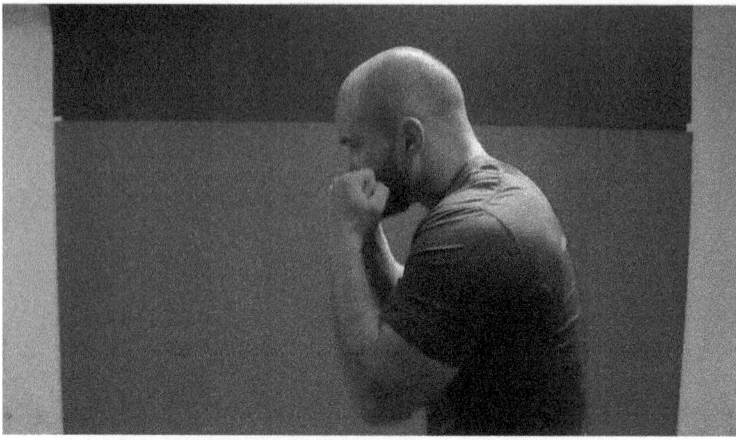

Figure 81: Return to start position.

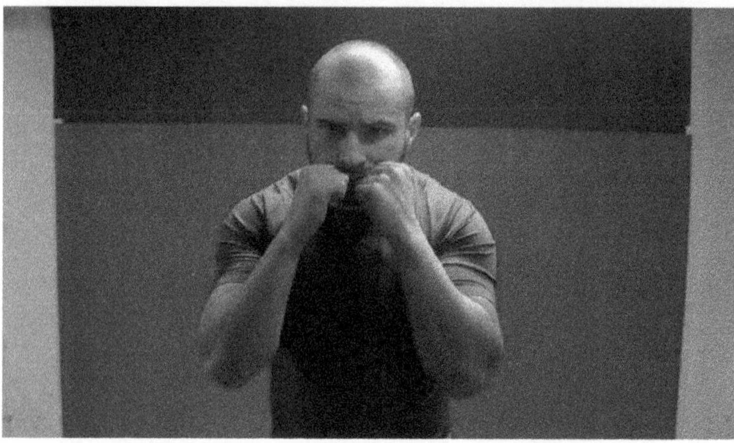

Figure 82: This is the front view of the cross.

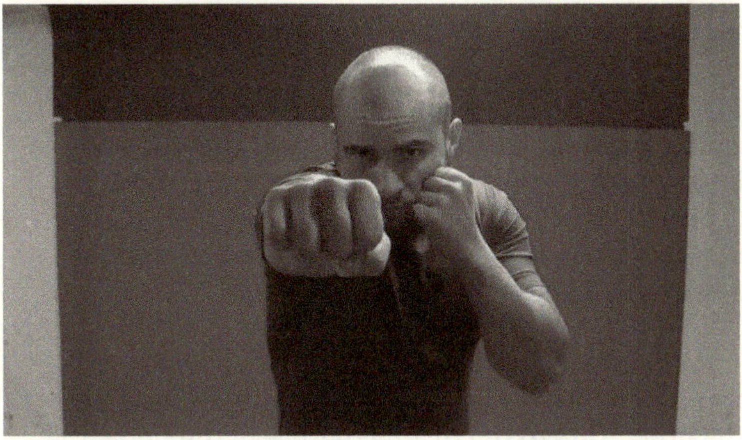

Figure 83: Throw the punch straight out.

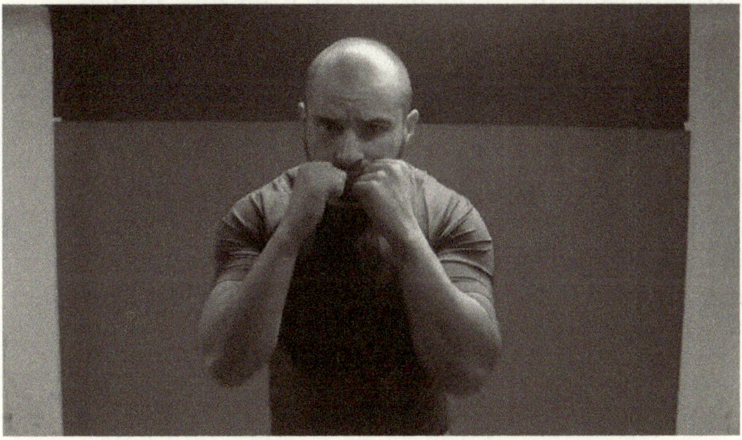

Figure 84: Return to start position.

The Hook

The hook is arguably the most powerful punch that can be thrown. The reason for this is that the body can be torqued in order to deliver more power. This is especially true with the rear hook. Due to the greater distance from target, the rear hook can gain more momentum and deliver more damage.

All punches use some form of hip drive and trunk rotation to deliver power. This is most applicable to the hook. Due to the turning nature of the hook, the hips and trunk are able to rotate which results in greater power output. This power is transferred into the target and can cause more damage when properly applied. Where the jab will generally cause damage through repetition, the hook can offer one-punch knockout power.

All punches require correct technique for optimal results. This is truer with the hook. The shoulder, elbow, wrist, hips, knees, and all need to rotate in proper alignment for maximum power. Without this technique, power is lost and a person can become unbalanced in the movement, which leaves them open to attacks. Let's look at the hook.

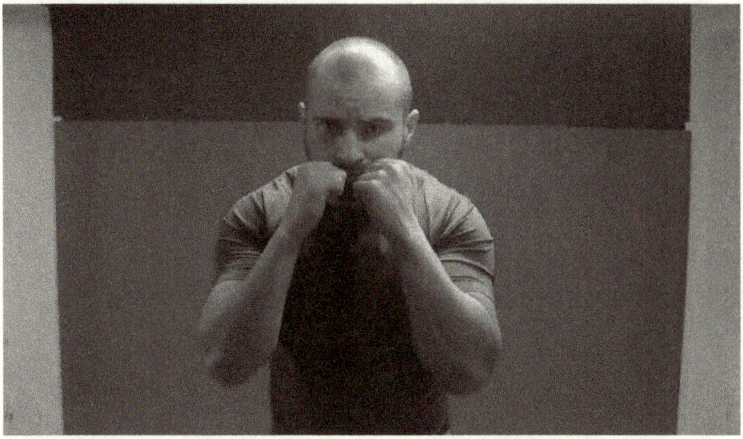

Figure 85: The hook starts from the standard stance.

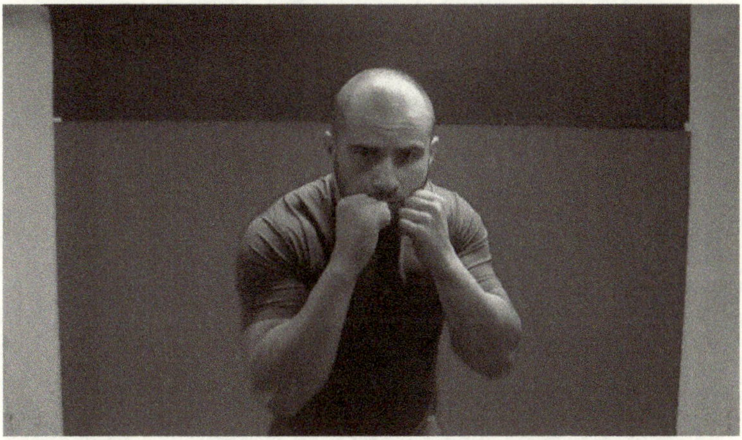

Figure 86: To throw the front hook, twist your body slightly toward the front arm. This torques the punch.

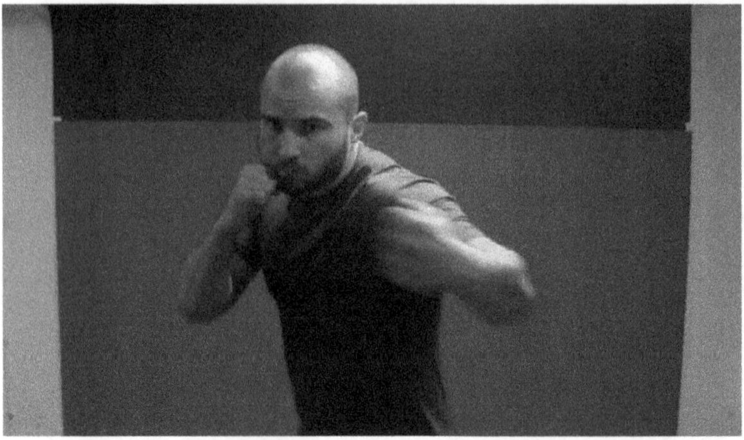

Figure 87: Rotate explosively out of this torque. The punch will travel in a circular motion toward the face (jaw line) of the attacker. This image shows mid punch.

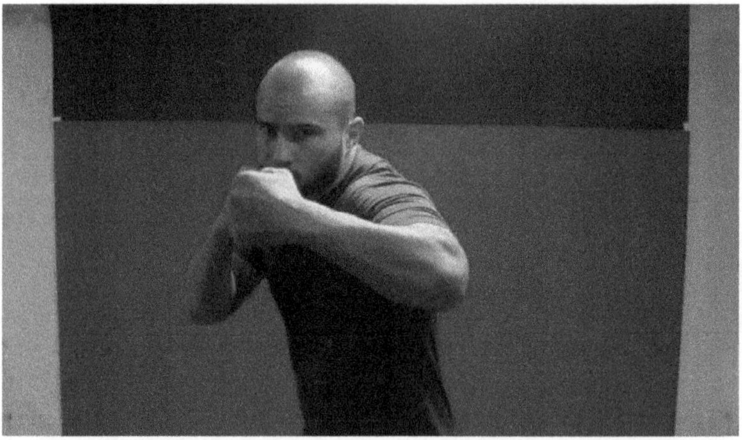

Figure 88: The punch stops once it has hit its target. If you miss, the elbow should not pass your face before returning your arm to the start position.

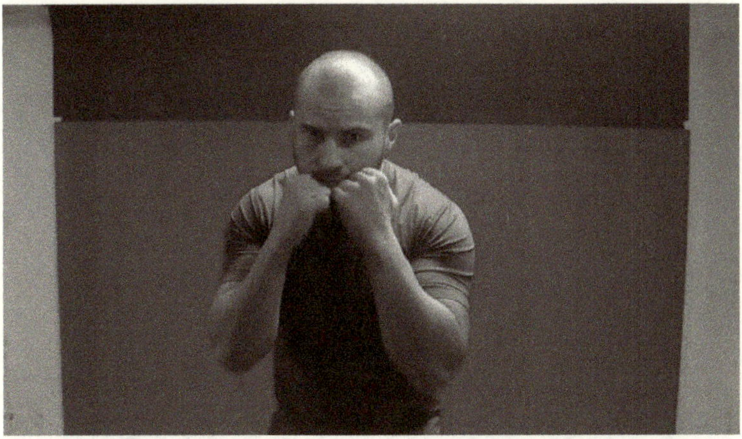

Figure 89: Return the punch to the start position. You can now throw the rear hook. It starts from the standard stance.

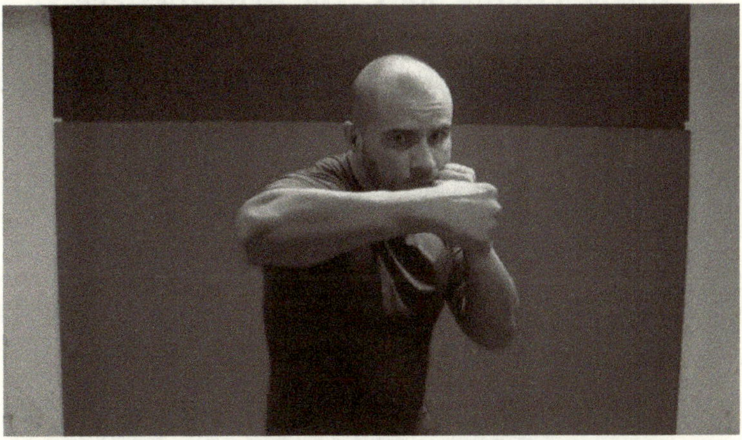

Figure 90: It travels in the exact same manner as the front hook. You will be able to achieve more rotation with the rear hook.

Hook to the Body

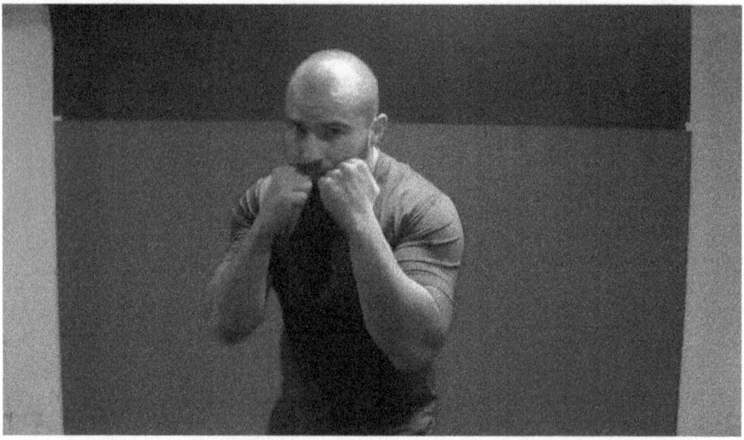

Figure 91: The front and rear hook can also be thrown to the body. The dynamics are generally the same. The main difference comes in the path that the punch travels.

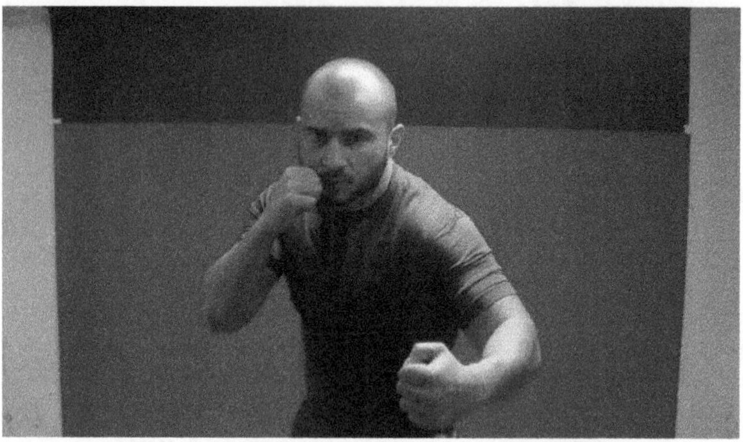

Figure 92: There is a downward angle with the rear hook to the body...

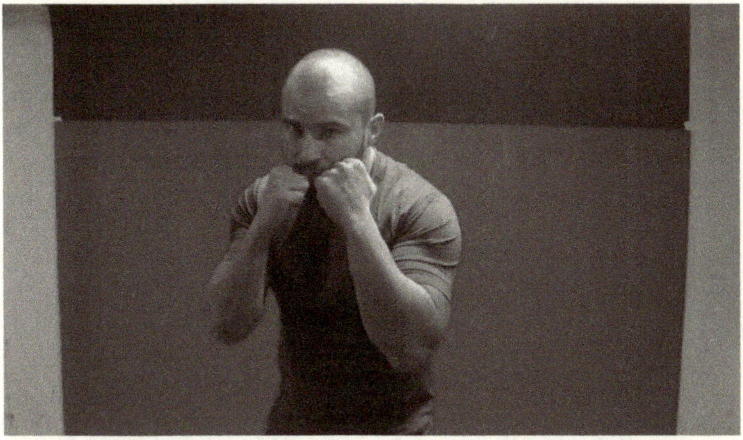

Figure 93: before it returns to the start position. You can now throw the rear body shot...

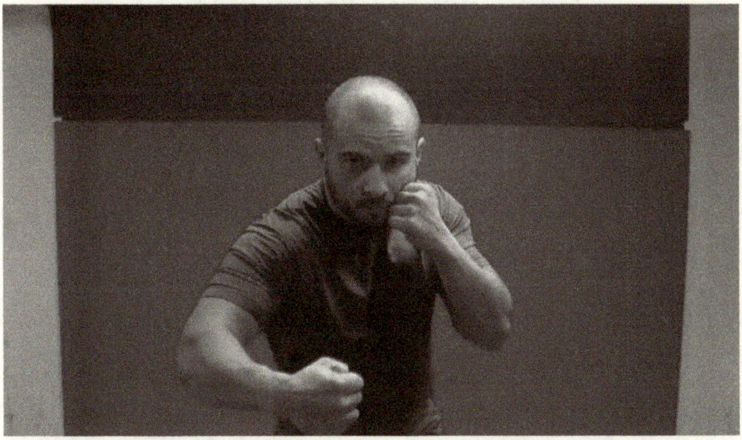

Figure 94: which travels with the same downward trajectory. Return to the start position.

The Uppercut

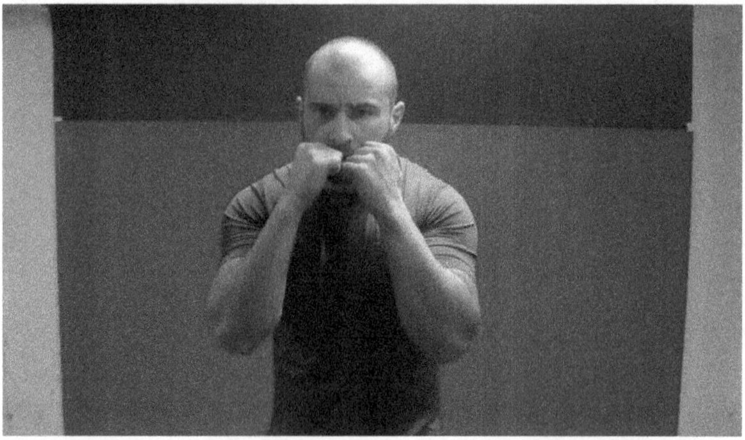

Figure 95: The uppercut works in much the same manner as the hook.

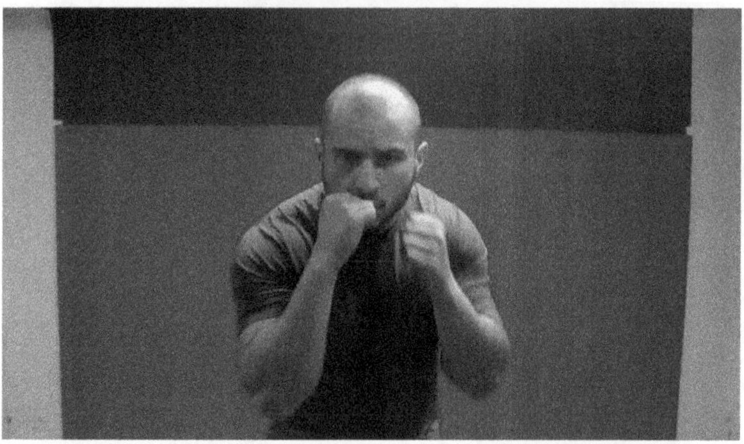

Figure 96: You will torque your body toward the side of you front hand when throwing the front uppercut.

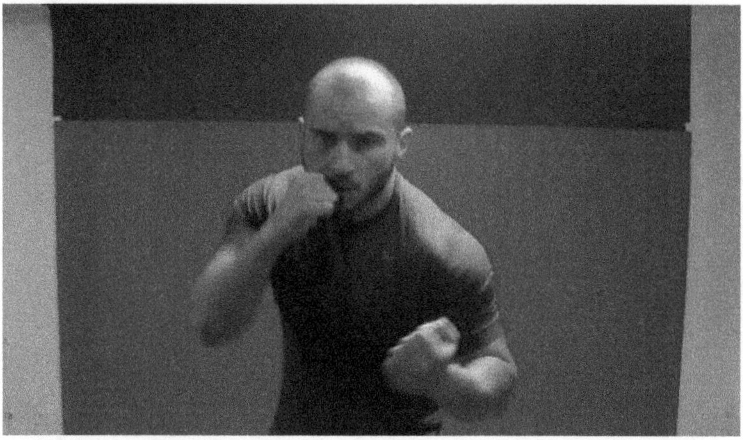

Figure 97: It will travel at an upward angle toward the head (instead of across like the hook)

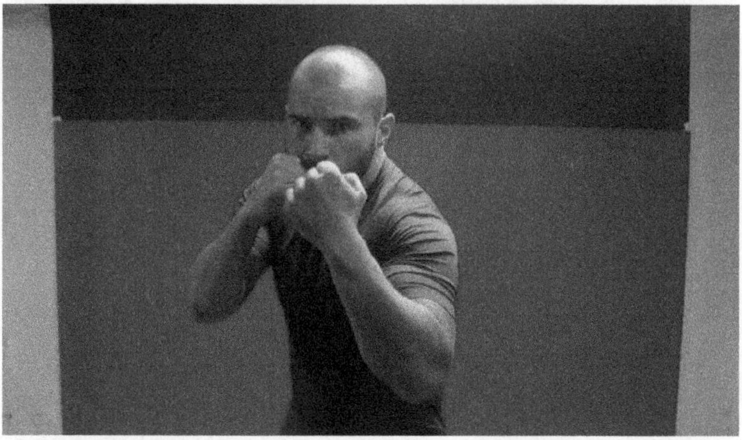

Figure 98: The punch ends when connection to the target is achieved. If you miss, do not let the elbow pass your face.

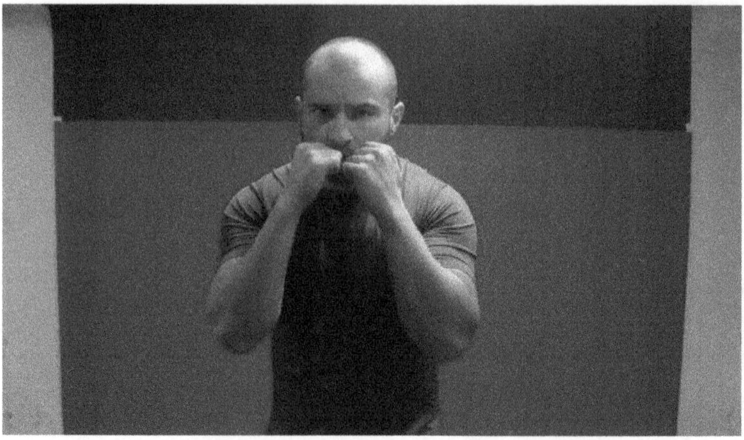

Figure 99: Return to start position. You can now throw the rear uppercut.

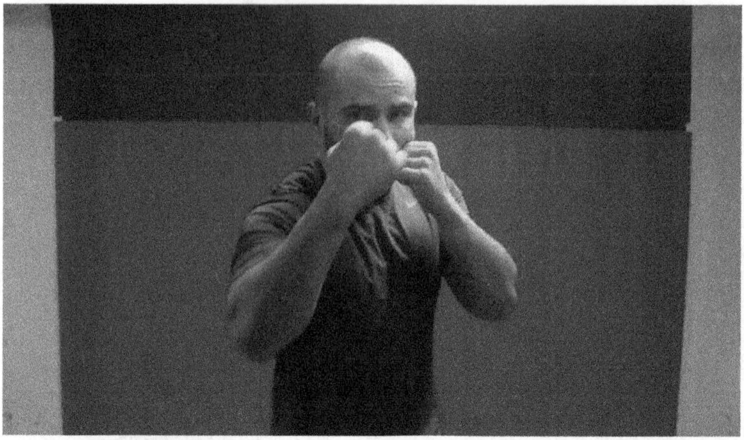

Figure 100: It moves in the same manner as the front hook, except there will be more rotation (similar to the rear hook).

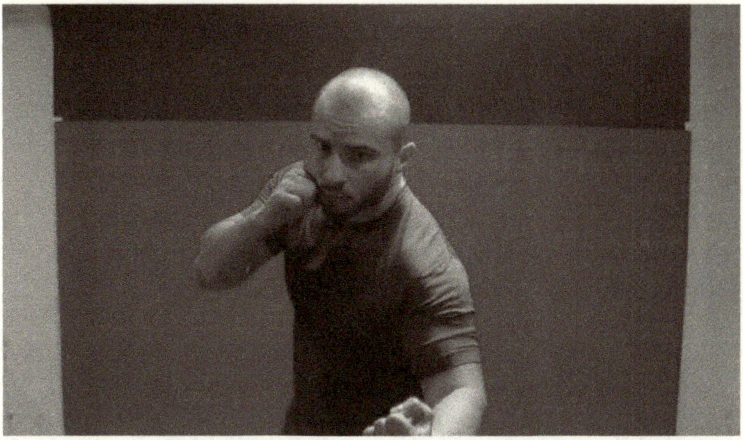

Figure 101: The front and rear uppercuts can also be thrown to the body. Similar to the hooks to the body, the uppercut to the body will simply travel a lower path. This shows the body uppercut.

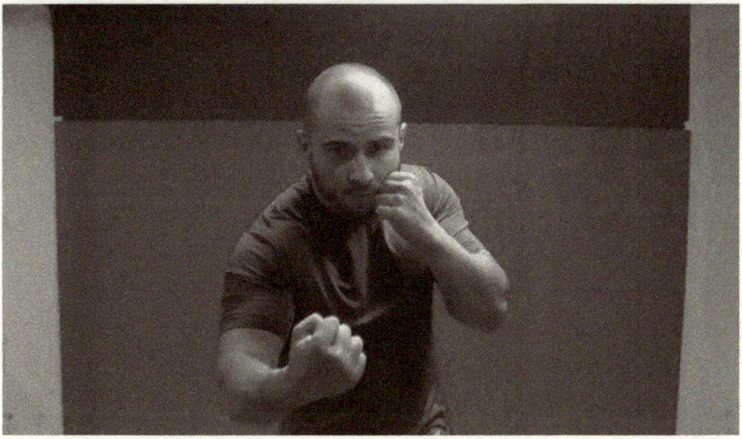

Figure 102: A shot of the rear body uppercut.

The 1-2 and the #6 Combo

Once you have learned the basic punches as individual moves, you can start putting them together in combos. A combo is simply a series of strikes, in this case punches, thrown in succession. The **1-2 Combo** is the basic combo learned with punches. It is the jab followed by the cross. Here is an example:

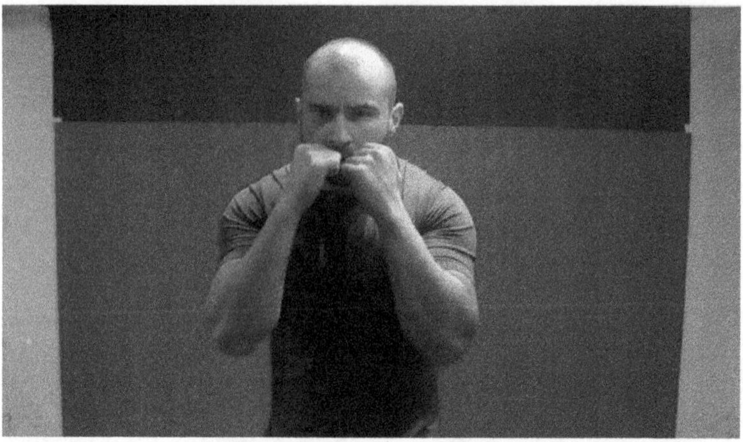

Figure 103: The 1-2 Combos start for the basic stance.

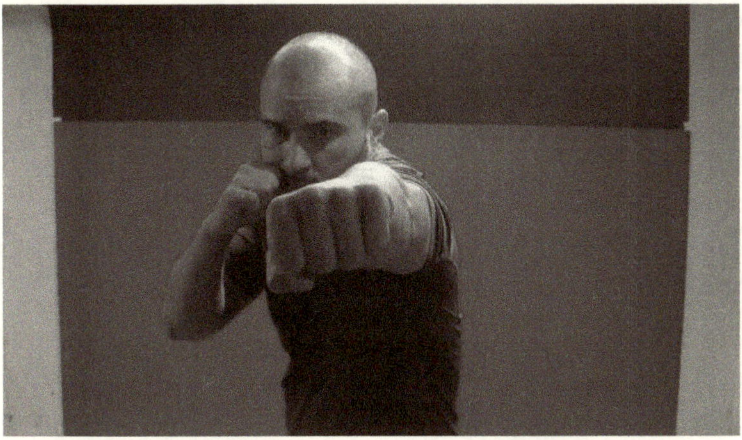

Figure 104: Throw the jab.

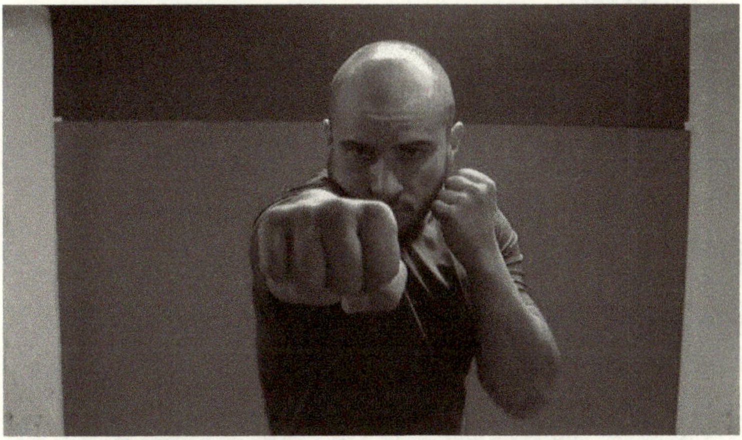

Figure 105: As the jab is returning you throw the cross. Then you return both hands to the start position. It's essentially that simple, but will take practice to perfect.

The **#6** combo is a series of six punches chained together. It focuses on using the torque created from each punch to set up the next punch. For example, when you throw the jab, you torque the body so that it is primed to throw the cross. When you throw the front hook, you torque the body so that it is primed to throw the rear hook. Think of it as elastic buildup. When you throw one punch, the muscles on that side elongate while the muscles on the other side shorten. This shortening causes a buildup of energy that can be utilized.

Working with that principle in mind, you will now learn the **#6** combo. The combination consists of the following punch order:

1. Jab,
2. Cross,
3. Front hook,
4. Rear hook,
5. Front uppercut, and
6. Rear uppercut.

After the last punch is thrown, you reset to the start position with your hands high.

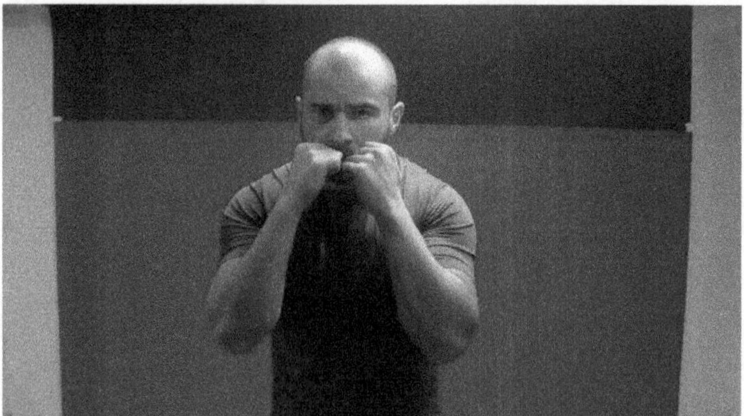

Figure 106: This is the start position for the #6 combo. It is your normal staggered stance.

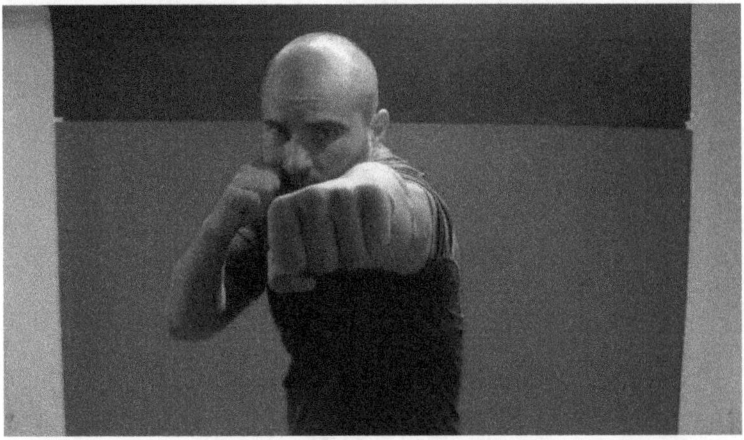

Figure 107: You throw the jab. As you are pulling the jab back...

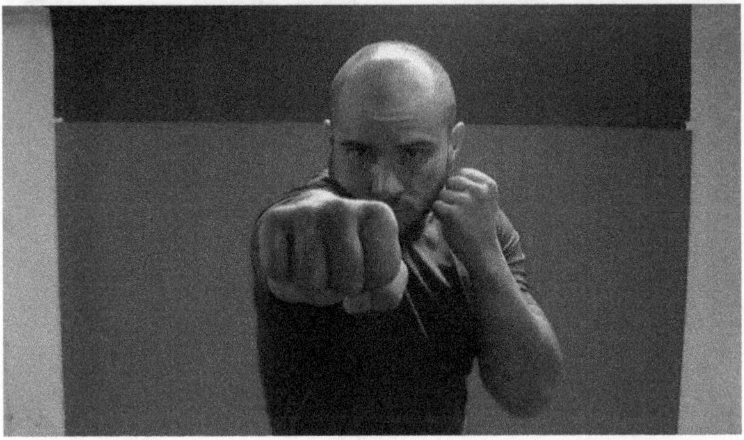

Figure 108: You throw the cross. As the cross is coming back...

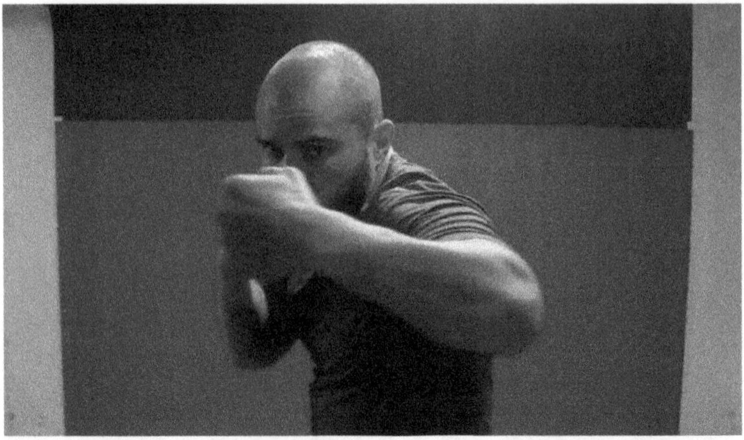

Figure 109: you throw the front hook. As the front hook is coming back...

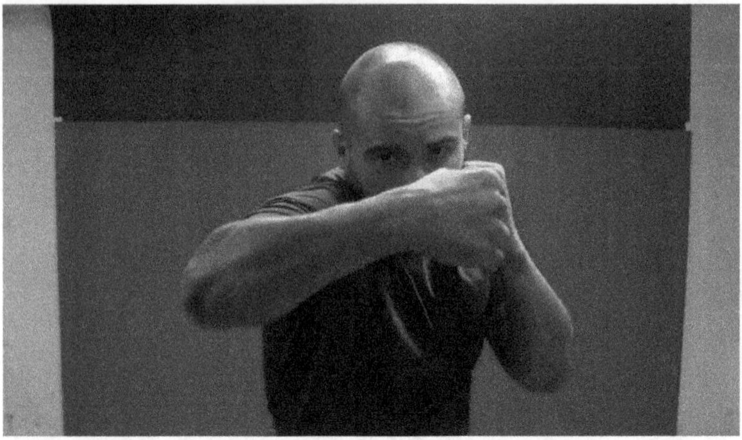

Figure 110: you throw the rear hook. As the rear hook is coming back...

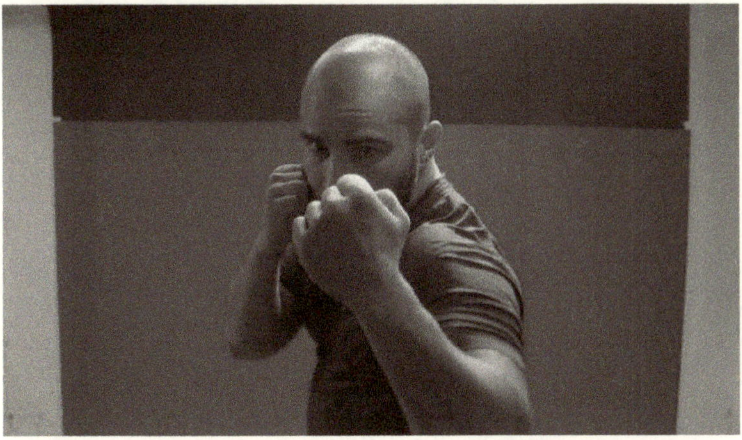

Figure 111: yu throw the front uppercut. As the front uppercut is coming back...

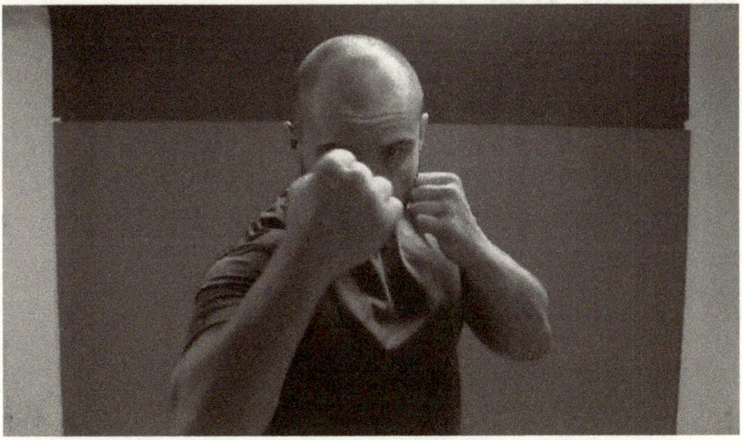

Figure 112: you throw the rear uppercut.

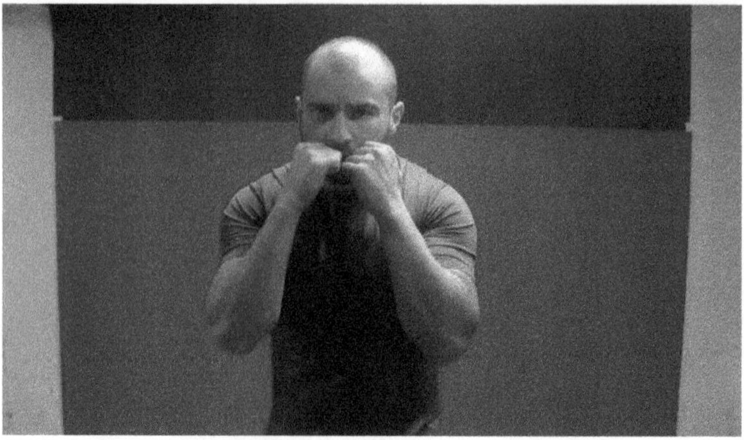

Figure 113: Return to start position.

Chapter Review

In this chapter, you have learned how to throw the six basic punches that are used in boxing and kickboxing. These are the jab, cross, front hook, rear hook, front uppercut, and rear uppercut. Mastering these will be key to the boxing portion of kickboxing.

Practice Suggestions

- Start the learning process by practicing each punch individually. Then practice two together, then three, and so on.
- Use a predetermined rep range. 5, 10, 15, or 20 for learning the punches. For example, do 10 jabs followed by 10 crosses.

- Once you are comfortable with one punch, start comboing. Work up to the #6 combo. Try mixing up the combinations as you get more comfortable.

Chapter 4: Basic Elbow and Knee Attacks

Elbow and knees strikes are just as they sound. When performing an elbow strike you will hit the attacker with an elbow. When performing a knee strike, you will hit the attacker with a knee. When executed properly, elbow and knee strikes are the some of the most devastating strikes.

The elbow is devastating for a few reasons. The first is the rotating motion that occurs with most elbow movements, such as the round elbow. Similar to the hook, this adds body torque which increases the power of the elbow, albeit for less range than the hook. The second, and most devastating aspect of an elbow strike, is the contact made by the tip of the elbow. The tip, or point, of the elbow is sharp. Hitting an attacker with this point has a high likelihood of cutting the person open. Bone to soft skin can be terribly damaging.

The knee is devastating due to the hard kneecap combined with leg power. With few exceptions, the legs are the most powerful muscle group in the body. They can deliver more power per inch than a punch can. Put this power behind a hard object and the effect of a hit is magnified. A knee to can break ribs, crack an orbital socket, and knock a person out.

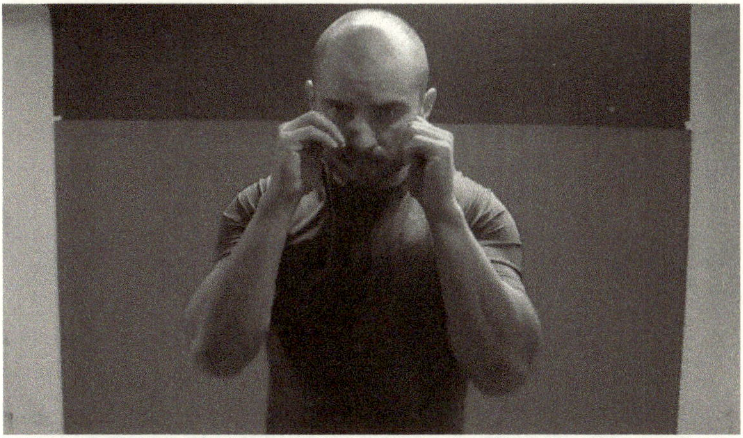

Figure 114: You are going to start with the basic round elbow. It is called the round elbow because it travels in half circle with a slightly upward trajectory. Start from your basic stance. When throwing an elbow, the hand should be open. Elbows can be thrown with a closed hand but the range of motion is limited and they are generally slower. Having the hand open allows you to tuck it close to your body.

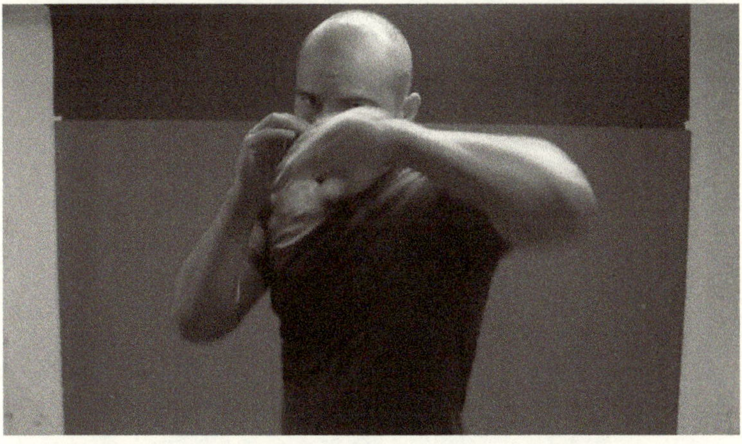

Figure 115: This image shows the front elbow in mid-strike. Notice that the elbow follows an upward trajectory. It has to follow this upward trajectory to achieve the top position needed to strike the face cross ways.

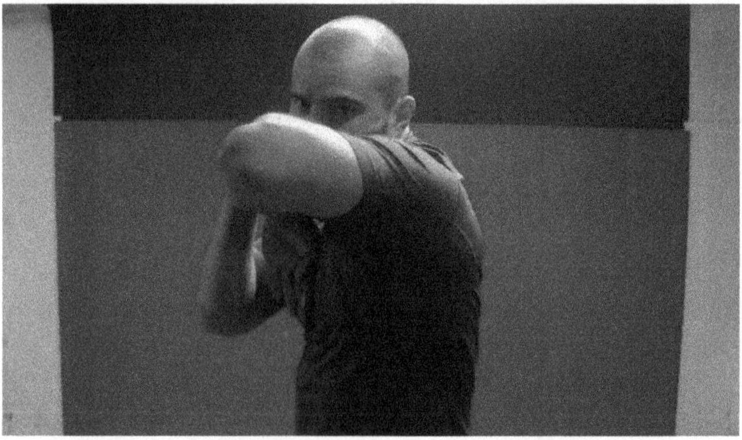

Figure 116: Once the elbow has reached the necessary striking level, it travels straight across the opponent's face. The pointy part of the elbow should strike the opponent. Notice how the hand on my striking arm is tucked in close to my chest. This is where the hand should stop.

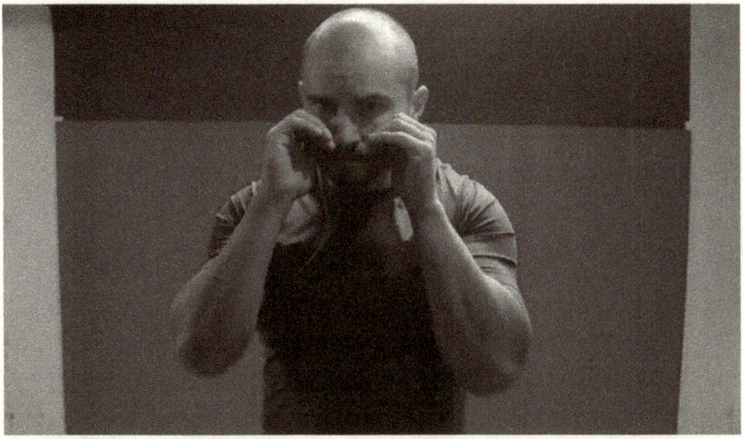

Figure 117: Return to start position. Repeat the same steps for the rear elbow. Like the rear hook, there will be more extension of the body. Refer to the rear hook for more details. You are now ready to throw the upward elbow.

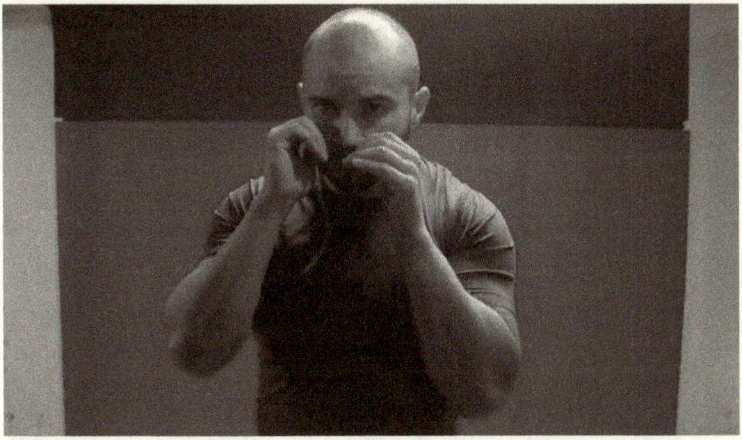

Figure 118: The upward elbow can start from the hands high position but it will have less momentum. To add more momentum, drop

the elbow slightly before throwing. This will be a bit of a tel, but when done quickly enough the elbow will still successfully hit the target.

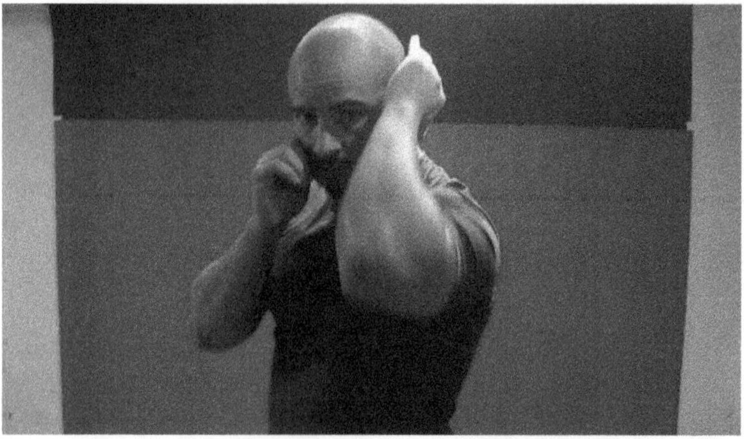

Figure 119: The upward elbow follows a straight trajectory moving skyward. You will strike the chin of the opponent.

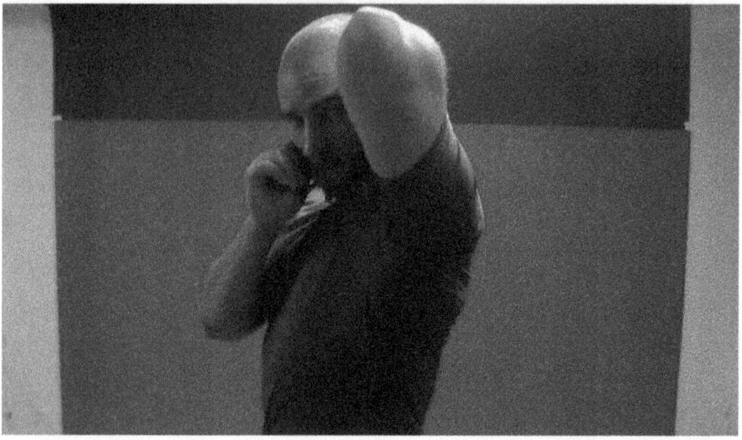

Figure 120: This is the fully extended position for the upward elbow. Notice that you are in a

very exposed position on the striking side. You do not want to stay in this extended position for too long.

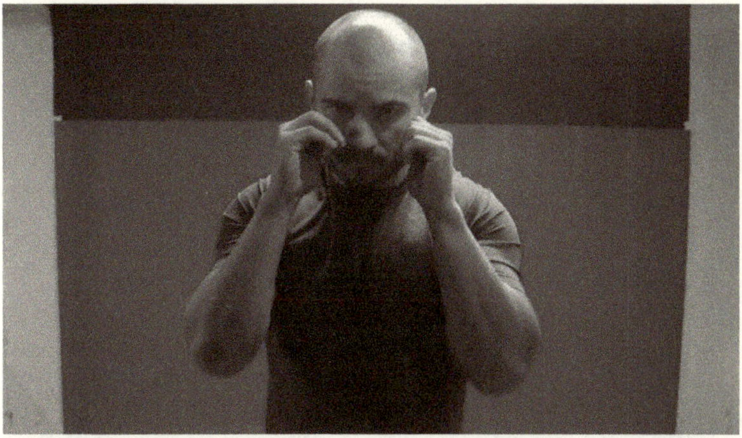

Figure 121: The next elbow you will learn is the downward elbow. The name is a bit misleading as the elbow actually comes downward with an inside angle. You will start from your standard stance.

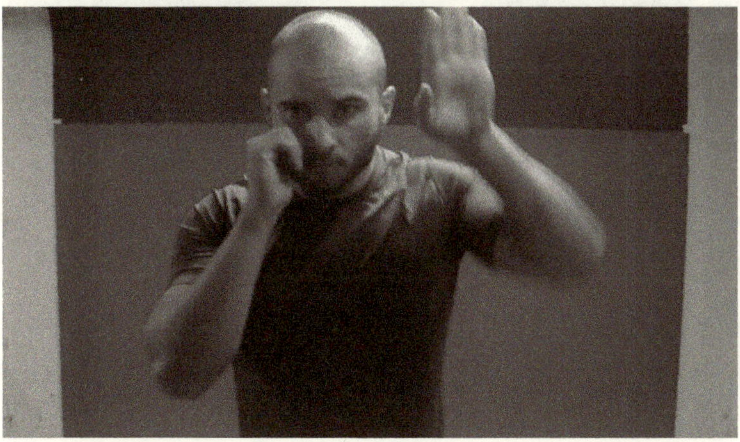

Figure 122: The elbow first travels in an upward circle motion. See the arrow. This motion is necessary to get the elbow to the appropriate height to perform the strike.

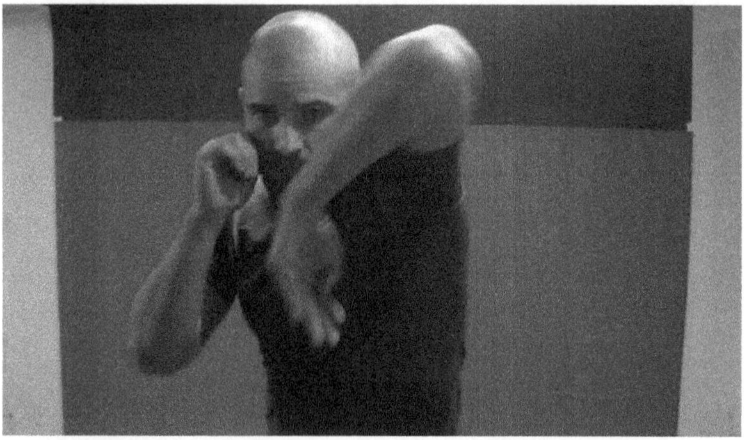

Figure 123: Once the elbow has achieved the necessary height it begins its downward trajectory.

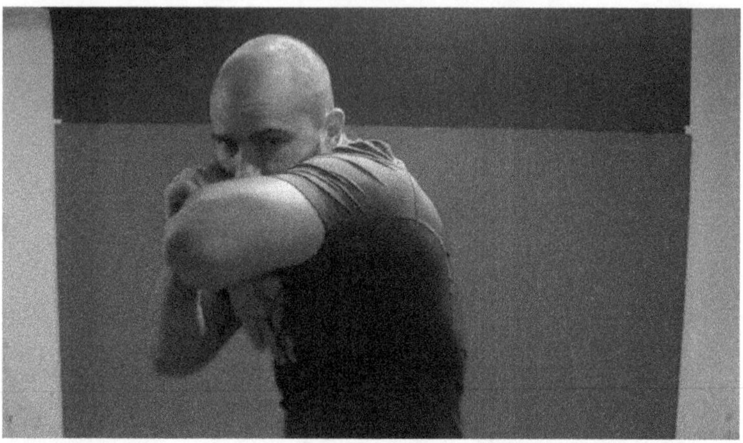

Figure 124: This image shows the elbow at the end of the strike. This attack is meant to come up and over the opponent's guard. It can be used to strike the opponent in the forehead, eye, or nose. This can lead to a broken nose, massive cut, or even a knockout blow. The blow follows the same path when thrown from the other side, again taking into consideration the greater range in motion.

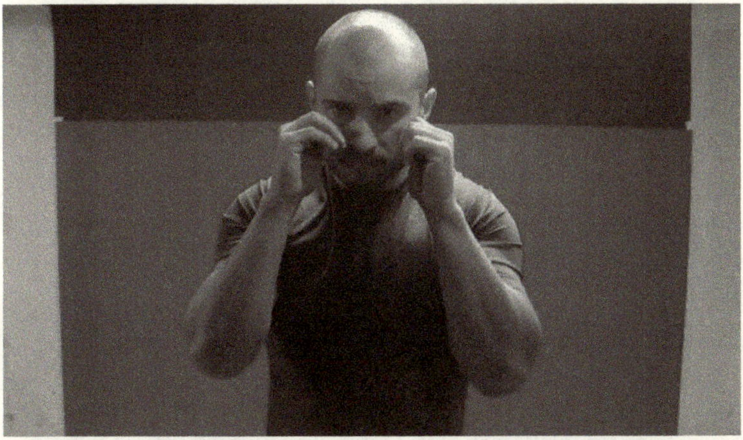

Figure 125: Return to the start position. You are now ready to throw the upward angle elbow. It travels in much the same manner as an upward elbow except this time it has an angle to it, similar in nature to the downward elbow.

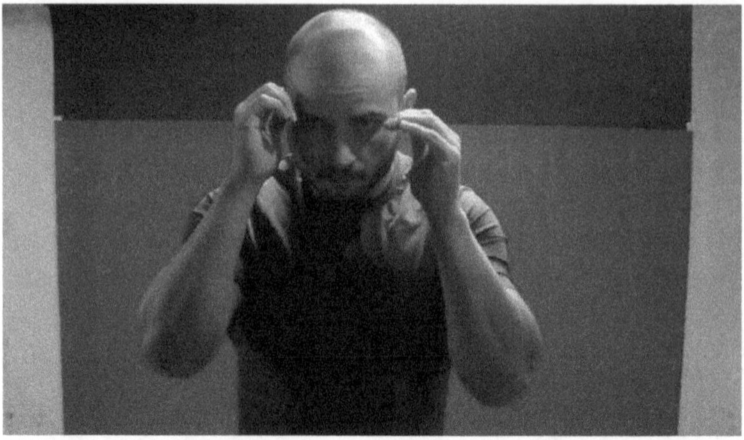

Figure 126: You will begin by dropping the elbow a few inches...

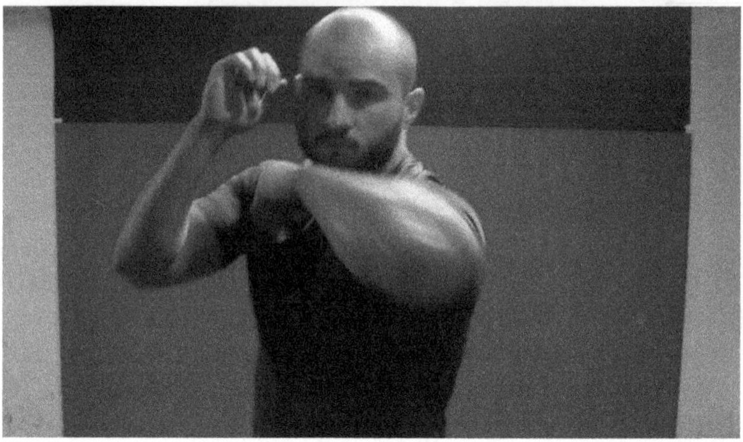

Figure 127: You will then begin driving it upward at an angle.

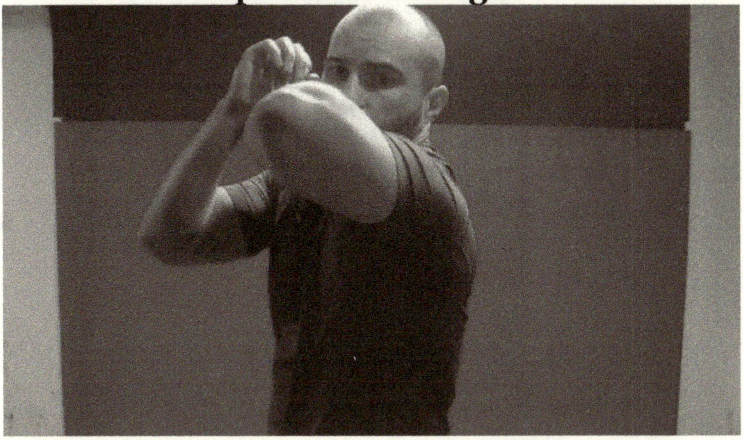

Figure 128: This is the top position for the elbow. You can extend a bit more than this but not too much. You expose yourself with this shot on both sides. You do not want to stay extended for long.

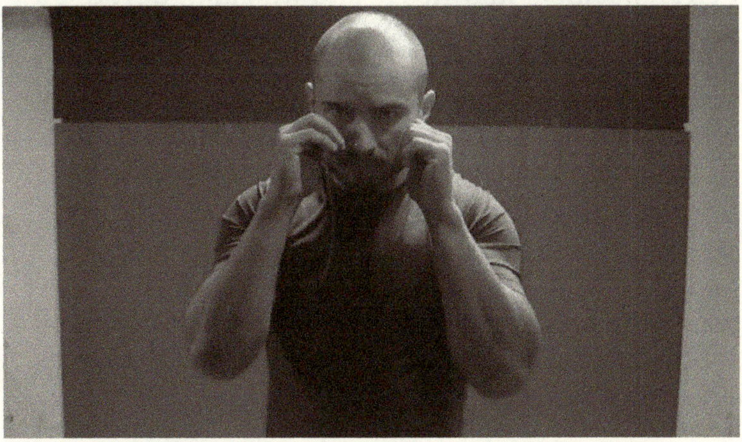

Figure 129: Return to start position.

Let's take a look at the following side shots for the elbows. As with the punches, you need to keep your hands high protecting yourself. Historically, when throwing elbows, a person would keep their non-striking hand open. Now this is a fine way to throw elbows. However, if you have been throwing punches then suddenly open your hands, a skilled opponent will be able to read that.

Now you might ask, how often am I going to run into a skilled opponent. Who knows? Maybe never. Maybe tomorrow. Why not train like everybody is skilled? The reason I say that is this, you never know what skill level a person has. Never underestimate anyone. They might surprise you.

Let me offer an example. I trained at a gym that offered a number of services including boxing and a weight training. Out in the weight training area I talked to a number of people. Over time I learned who was had combat knowledge and who didn't. At this gym, roughly 1 out of every 3 males had some form of combat knowledge. One out of three. With that in mind, let's train like everyone is skilled.

Keeping that thought in mind, let's look back at the elbows. Unless I am only training elbows, I like to keep my hands in fists. Punching is my primary weapon and so I want to stay with that hand positioning. With practice, I have become very adept at opening the striking hand right before I throw an elbow strike.

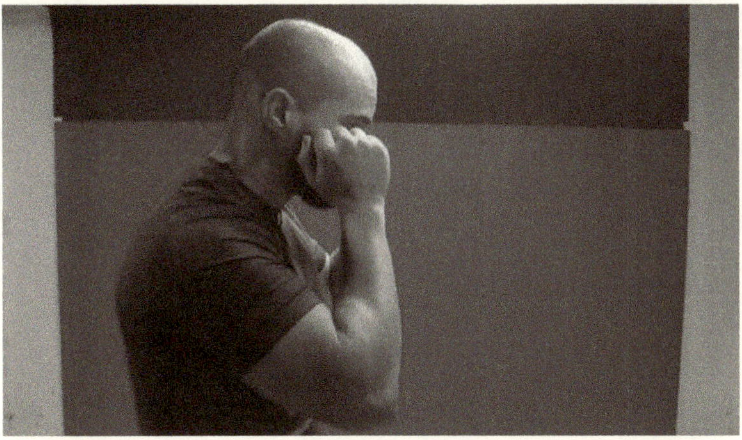

Figure 130: In this image, I am in my basic punching stance. My hands are tight to may face.

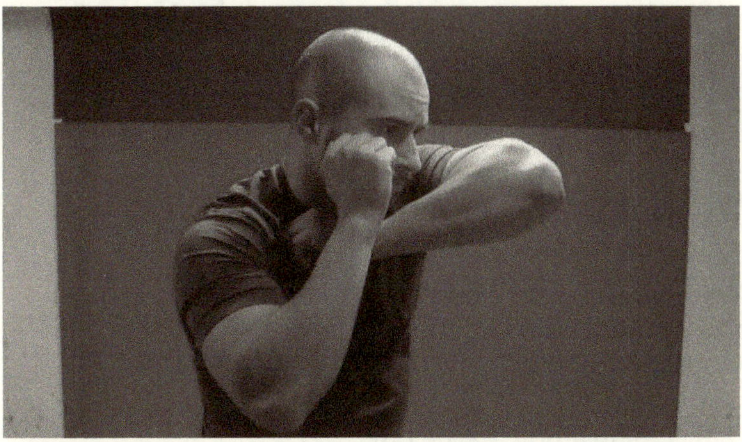

Figure 131: Right before I throw my elbow I allow my hand to open which facilitates the elbow strike. My non-striking hand is high to my face, in a fist.

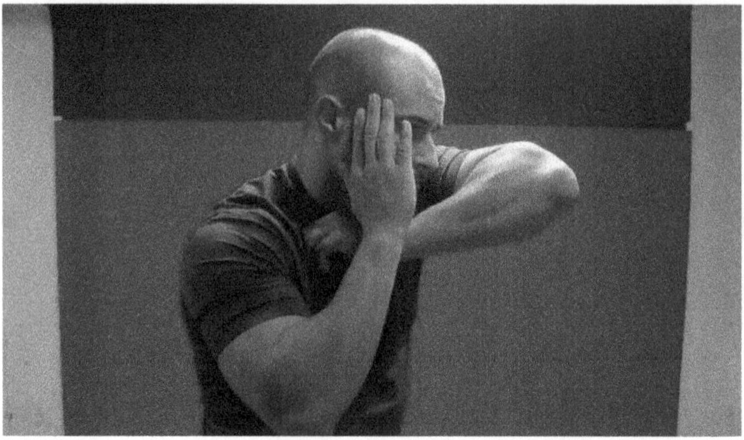

Figure 132: In this image, I am using the open palm version of defense. This is fine when training elbows only but, when working with punches and elbows, try to keep the hands closed and high to the face. Open the striking hand right before an elbow strike.

Rear Elbows

Rear elbows are elbows thrown behind the body. In this manual, you are going to be shown three variations:

1. The elbow to the gut,
2. The elbow to the chin, and
3. The elbow to the side of the head.

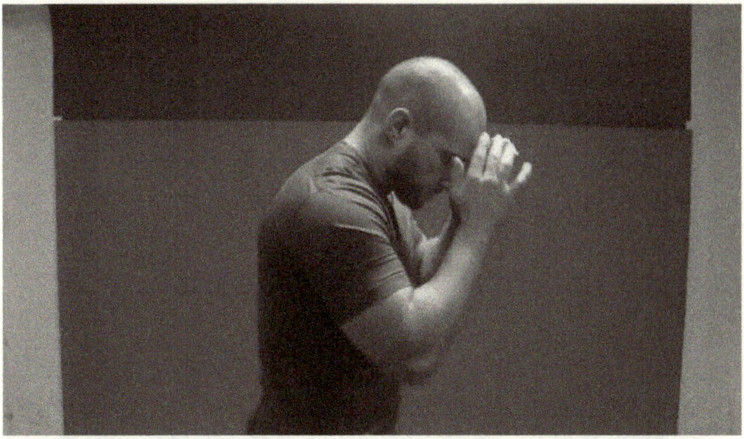

Figure 133: The elbow to the gut is not a powerful elbow, but it can hurt. When properly placed this elbow will hit a person in the solar plexus (diaphragm) and cause the opponent to suck air. This can allow you to create space or set up a strike. It begins with a forward stance.

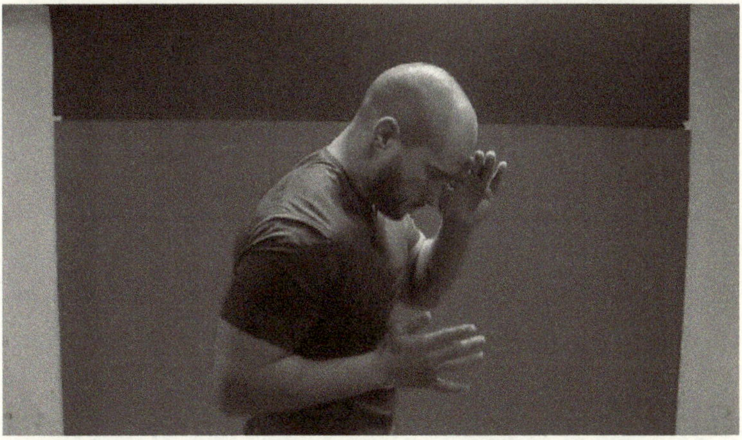

Figure 134: To perform this elbow you simply shove your elbow down and back in an arcing

or semi-circular motion. You then return it to the start position.

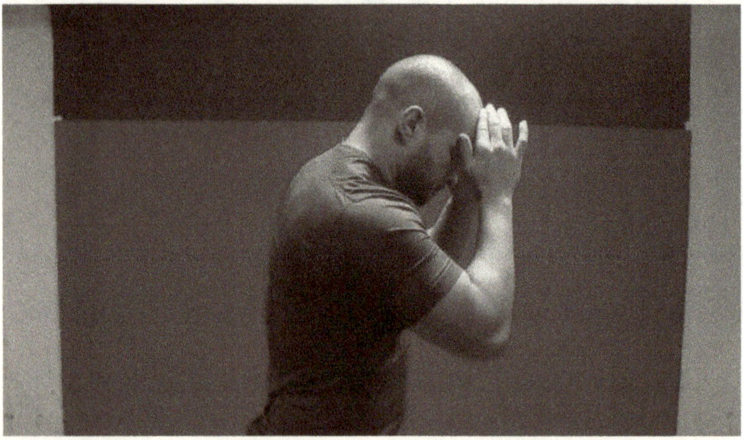

Figure 135: The next elbow is the rear elbow to the chin. It is delivered in much the same manner as the rear elbow to the gut. The difference lies in the range of motion and the need to lean forward slightly to facilitate full range of motion.

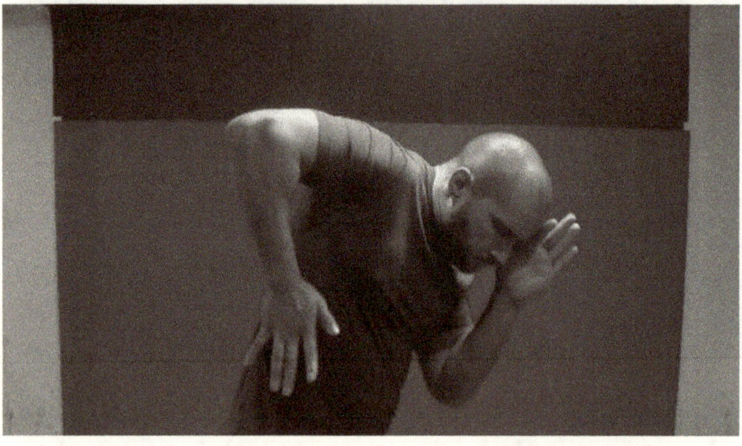

Figure 136: Start from a guard position. Drive your elbow down and back in an arcing or half-circle motion. As you do this, you will need to lean slightly forward. How far will be indicated by your height in comparison to the person you want to strike, and your flexibility. Stop the movement when you hit the person's jaw, or the imagined position of the person's jaw. Return to start position.

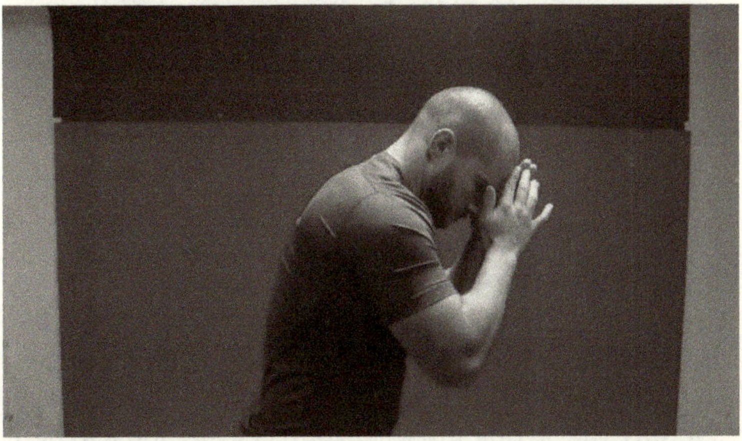

Figure 137: The next elbow is a round elbow to the side of the head. It travels in an upward round angle. Ideally, you will strike the opponent on the side of the head by the jaw or temple. Depending on exact distance from opponent and angle, it could vary. Start from the guard position. Your body will turn into the strike.

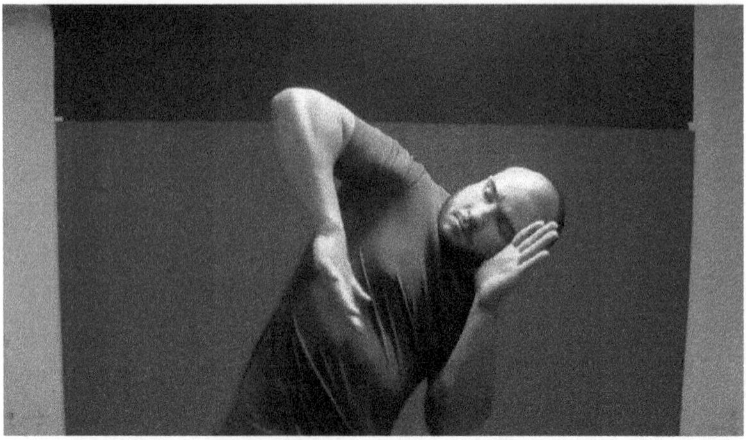

Figure 138: Your body will turn into the strike.

Knee Strikes

Knee strikes can be devastating attacks. The kneecap is a hard and relatively immobile surface. The legs are generally the strong muscle groups in the body. When the power of the leg is put against the kneecap it can result in a knockout, broken ribs, a broken nose, and many other injuries.

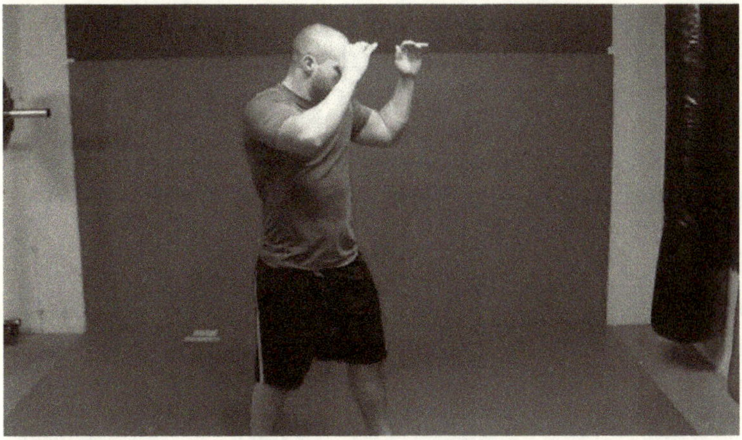

Figure 139: The forward knee strike is the most basic knee strike. This strike is done form a standard stance. In the image, my hands and arms are slightly more apart than normal. This is easier for me when throwing knees and kicks. The knee travels in a forward-upward angle.

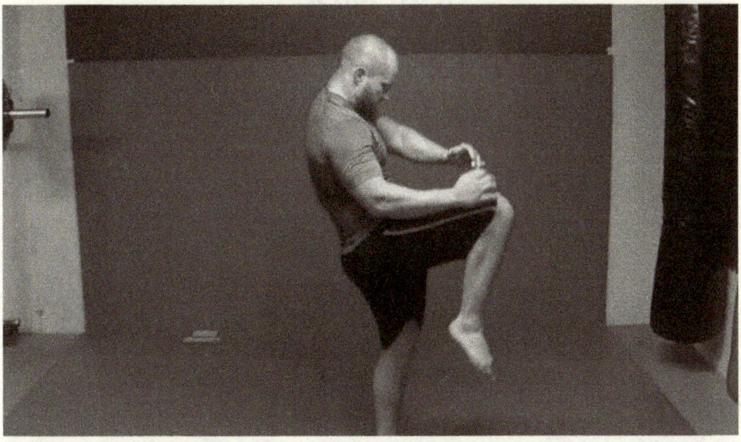

Figure 140: This knee strike is often thrown from the clinch via head grab. You pull the

person's head down as you throw the knee upward. I am mimicking this in the image. This shot, when properly performed, is a knockout shot.

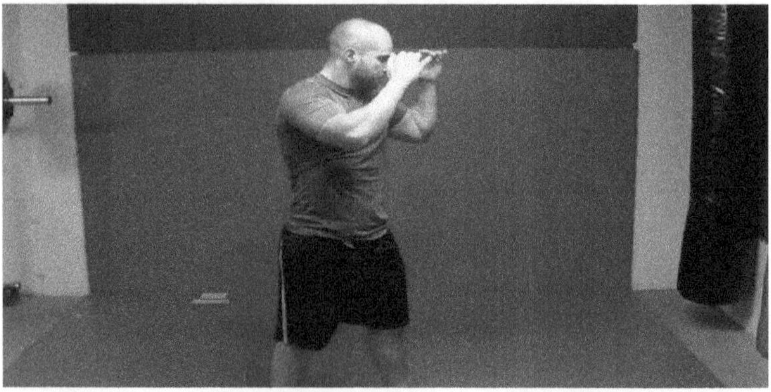

Figure 141: The forward knee can be thrown without the clinch as well. The motion will be basically the same as the previous version. The differences will be no head grab and a slight lean back.

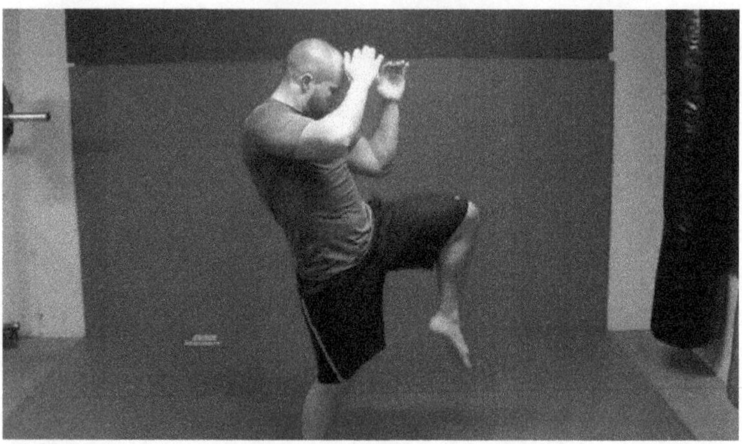

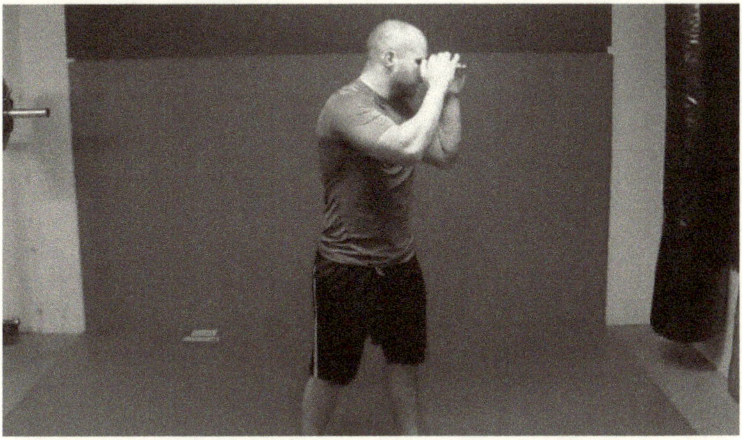

Figure 142: Either knee can come with or without the clinch.

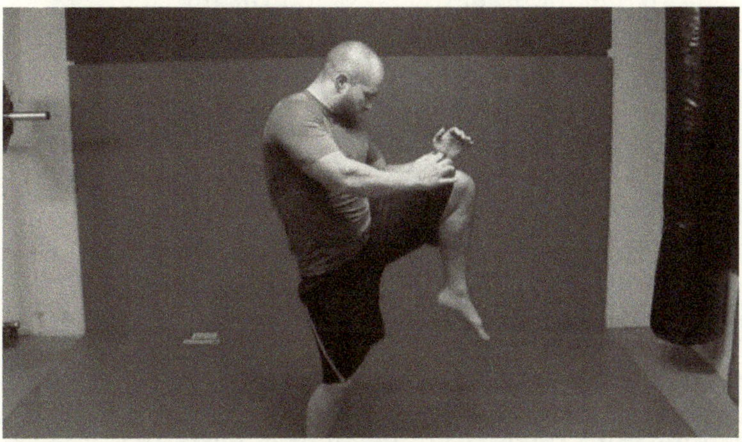

Figure 143: Attempt throwing both clinch and non-clinch version with both knees.

Chapter 5: Basic Kick Attacks and Defense

Attacking with kicks is an art unto itself. Every able-bodied person on Earth has the ability to perform a kick and has kicked something in their life. However, just because someone has kicked a ball or a heavy bag, it does not mean that the kick was done correctly. In kicking sports and martial arts that incorporate kicks, there is a specific technique with which to kick in order to achieve maximum efficiency.

In sports such as football or soccer, the kicker has to strike the ball with their foot using ideal technique to achieve maximum power, which turns into ball velocity. This same idea is applied to martial arts except this time the goal is maximum impact on a target. Speed and power are needed for both sports based kicking and martial arts based kicking. This does not mean that a larger, stronger person is going to be the more powerful kicker. To be a powerful kicker, this speed and power must be focused in proper technique. It is in this way that a smaller person can deliver a more powerful kick than a larger person.

Let me offer you an example of differences in power that are not based on size, but rather on years of technique practice. I have been using kick strikes for about three years now. A gentleman I know has been using kick strikes for close to thirteen years. He weighs around 140 pounds while I walk around at roughly 195 pounds. We both use the Bob heavy bag in our training. Bob weighs approximately 270 pounds with a full base. I have good technique so when I deliver a roundhouse kick I can almost knock Bob over. This other gentleman, the one that weighs roughly 140 pounds, can kick Bob over completely.

Now, do not let that example be intimidating to you. The gentleman I am referencing is a black belt in Tae Kwon Do and has trained Muay Thai in Thailand. He breathes martial arts. My point with that example is to stress the importance of correct technique. You should not expect to ever be perfect, let alone to be perfect quickly. With time and practice, you will become proficient in all the techniques exampled here, including the round kick. When I first started training Muay Thai, I could barely make a heavy bag move. With practice, I've become better.

The Teep

The teep is a type of front kick. It is also known as the foot-jab or push-kick. The kick is historically considered a defensive kick. It is used to push an opponent away from you. This can be used to set up other strikes as well. For example, you can push-kick an opponent from you to create distance and then deliver a round kick. The following series of images will illustrate the teep.

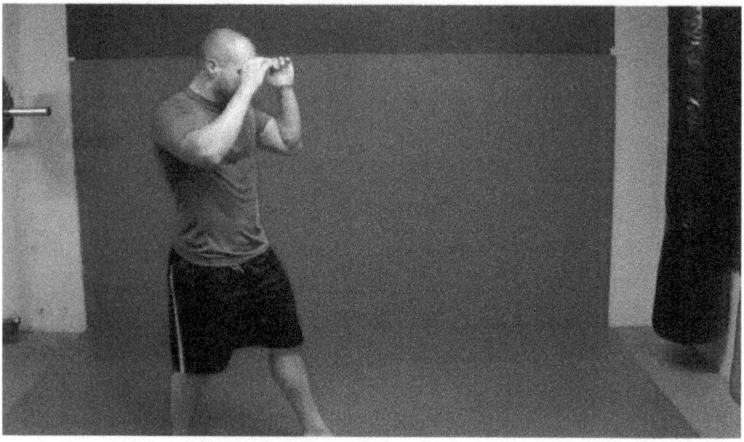

Figure 144: To complete the teep, you start by bringing the knee up. We will start with the back leg.

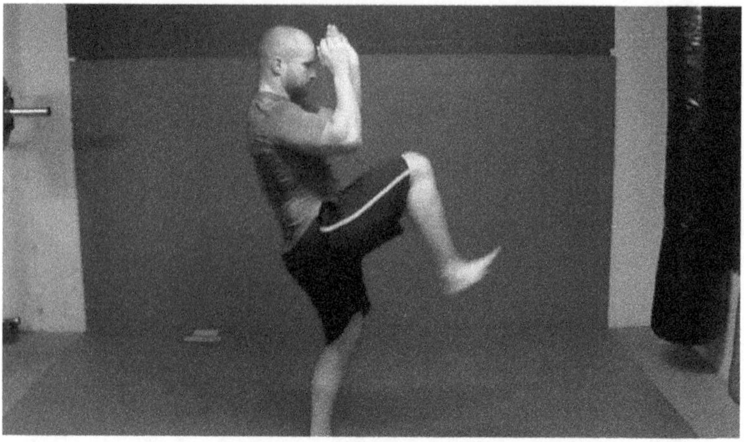

Figure 145: Bring the knee up to above waist height. You will lean slightly back while balancing on the non-kicking leg. From this position, you will kick straight out.

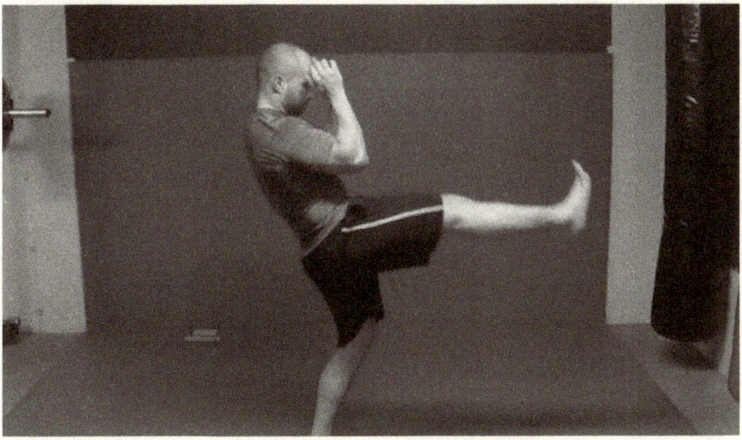

Figure 146: Kick your leg straight out. In this image, I am shadowboxing, but if faced with an opponent, I would target the gut area.

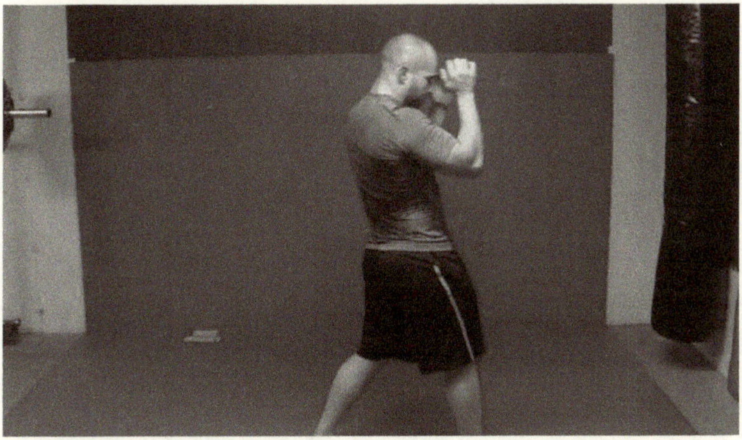

Figure 147: Your leg will come down as if finishing a forward step. You will be in a southpaw stance. Return to your normal stance.

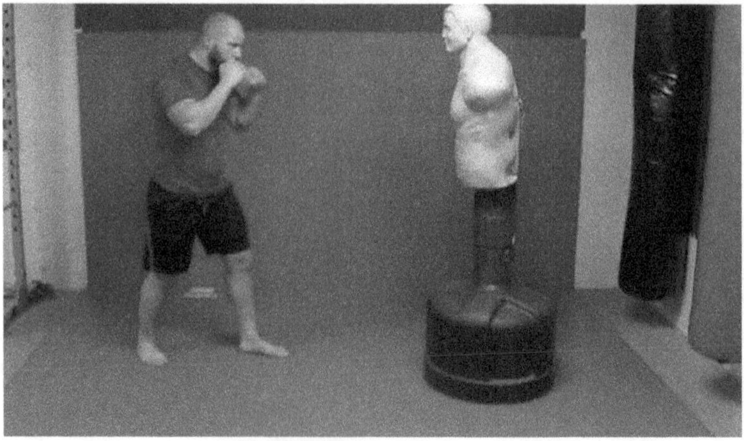

Figure 148: This is the rear teep on the punching Bob dummy. This is the start position.

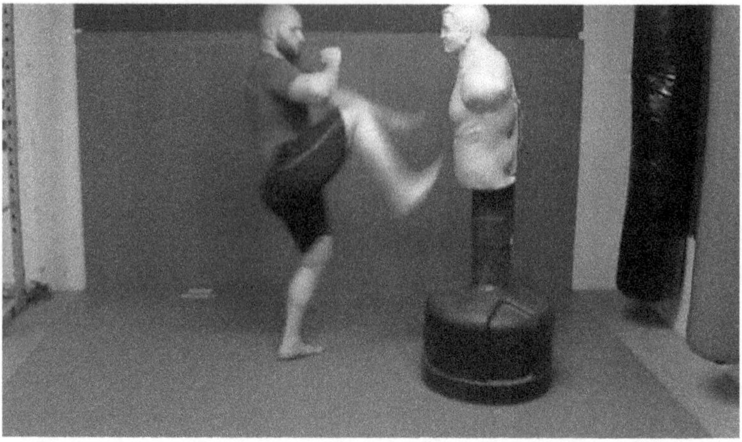

Figure 149: The leg is up high and ready to kick.

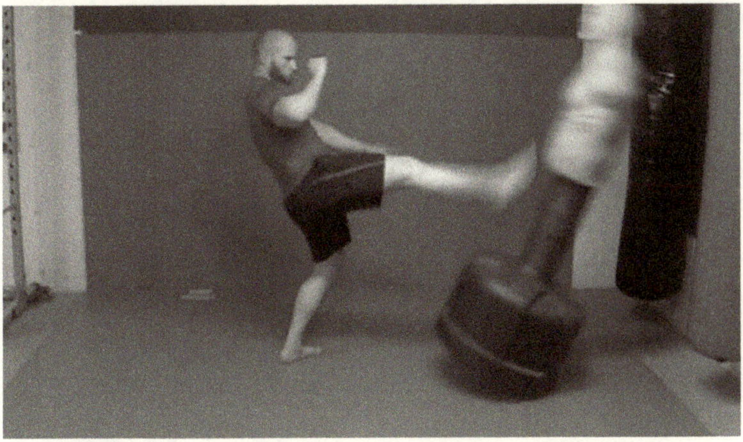

Figure 150: The extension of the kick.

Side Kick

The sidekick is essentially how it sounds. This kick is delivered from the side stance we reviewed earlier. The sidekick is an attacking kick that can be delivered to the legs, abdomen, and head. When properly applied this kick has serious power and can cause major damage to an opponent. For example, a sidekick delivered to the knee can snap the connective tissue supporting the knees and permanently handicap a person. The following is one variation of the side kick.

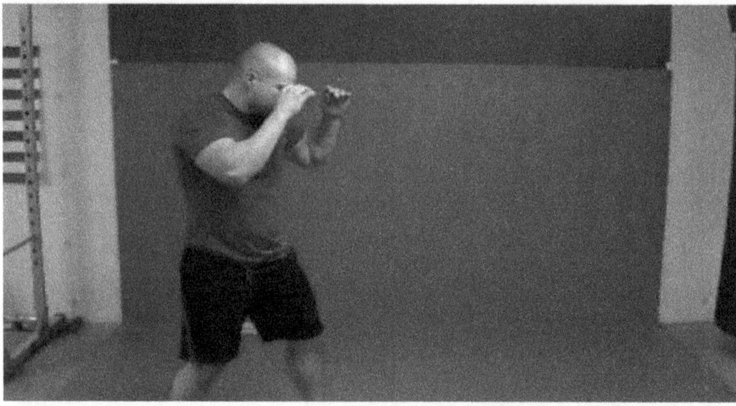

Figure 151: The basic sidekick is thrown from a side stance. This is the starting position. You will be throwing the kick with the back leg.

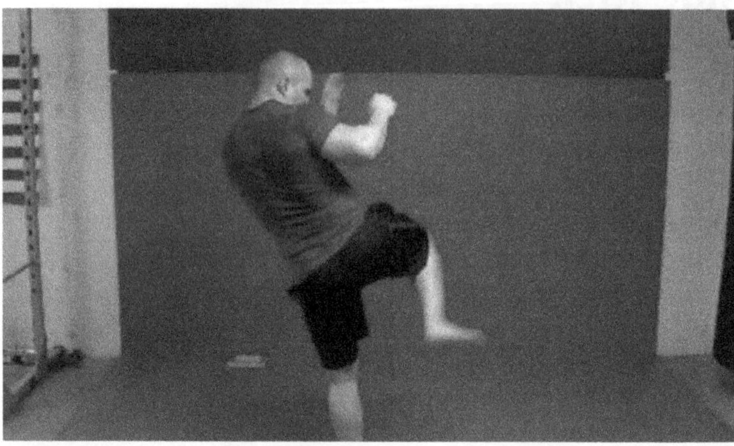

Figure 152: You start by bringing you rear leg forward and raising the knee. At the same time, you allow you non-kicking leg to rotate to facilitate the forward movement of the rear leg. The knee travels upward into the top

position for the side kick. Your hands stay high and protect the face as the leg is raised.

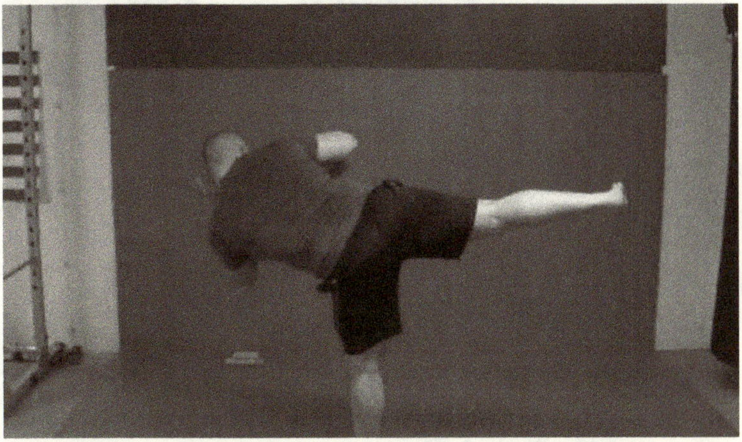

Figure 153: You then push the kick straight out from the body. You push from the hip of the kicking leg as well as the knee. You will have a lean back as you throw the kick. The rear hand stays high to the face and the front hand will drop down, as in the image.

The Basic Round Kick (Roundhouse Kick)

The basic round house kick is the staple of all kicking arts. It is the most commonly learned and executed kick across the board. Each style of martial arts, from karate to taekwondo, has its own variation of the round kick or roundhouse kick. In this guide, you will be shown what is commonly known as the Muay Thai style round kick.

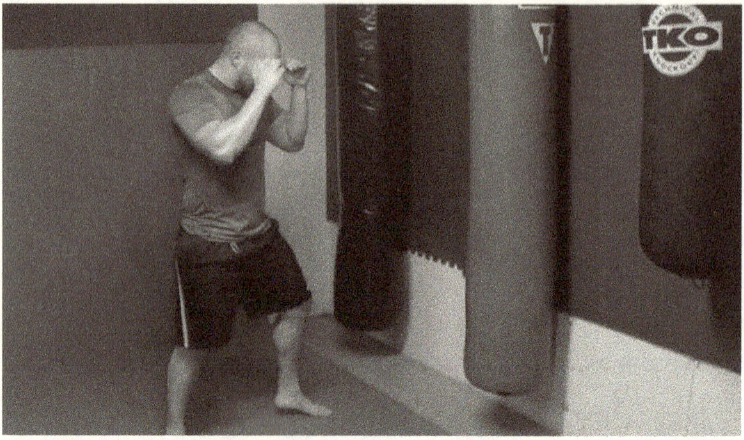

Figure 154: The round kick begins in the basic stance. Your hands may be a little looser than the boxing hand placement. By this, I mean they can be a little further from the face to allow for the necessary arm movement that accommodates the kick. From here you will throw a rear leg round kick. It will travel in an upward arching motion.

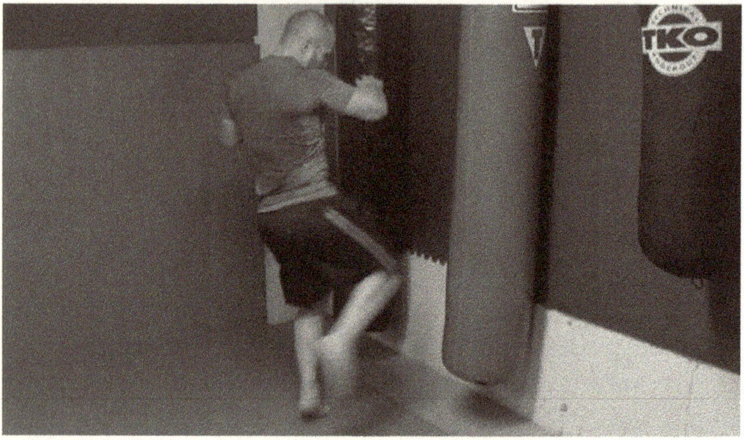

Figure 155: You pivot on your non-kicking leg to facilitate the rotation needed for the kick. At the same time, you allow your body to turn and your leg to lift from the ground and travel in the arching motion. Your kicking side hand will drop down as a counter-balance. Your hand on the non-kicking side stays tight to the face for protection.

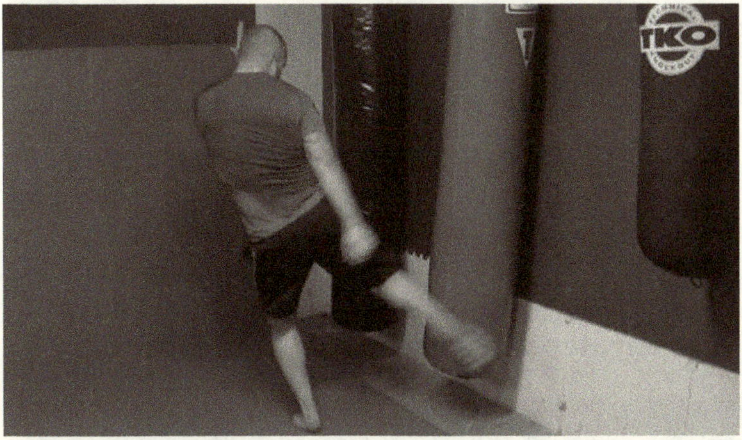

Figure 156: In this image, the kick is about to connect. Notice how my non-kicking foot is rotating at the ankle. Notice how may kicking side hand has dropped down. Notice that my far hand is tight by my face.

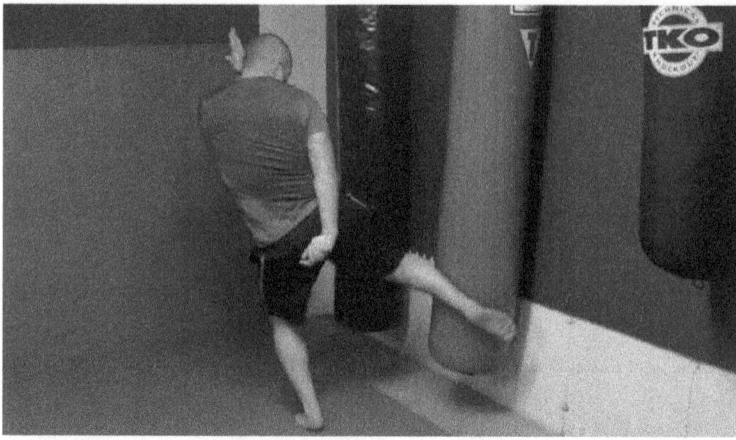

Figure 157: This is the completed kick. In this image, I have thrown a kick that would land at just above knee level of a person who is roughly 5"8" tall. Your kicking side hand does not need to be as far back as mine. I have exaggerated the movement slightly for effect.

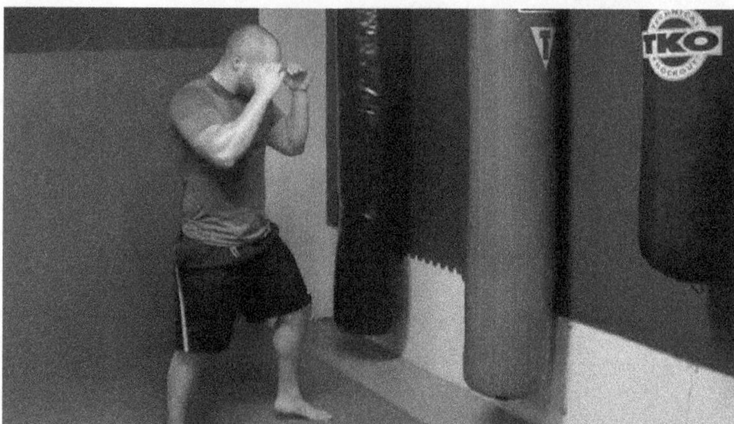

Figure 158: Return to start position. The path the leg and body travels backwards is the same

as it traveled when performing the forward motion of the kick.

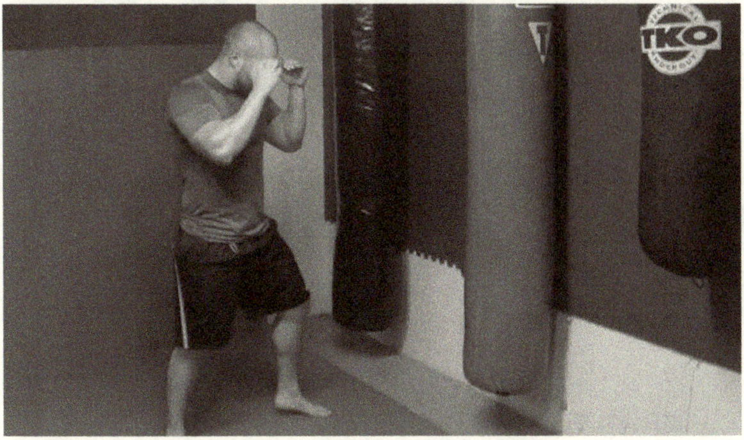

Figure 159: The round kick can be thrown to nearly any part of the body. This is of course dependent upon the striker's flexibility. An inflexible person will be limited in how high they can kick. In order to improve kicking height, improve flexibility along with technique. We are again at the start position for the round kick.

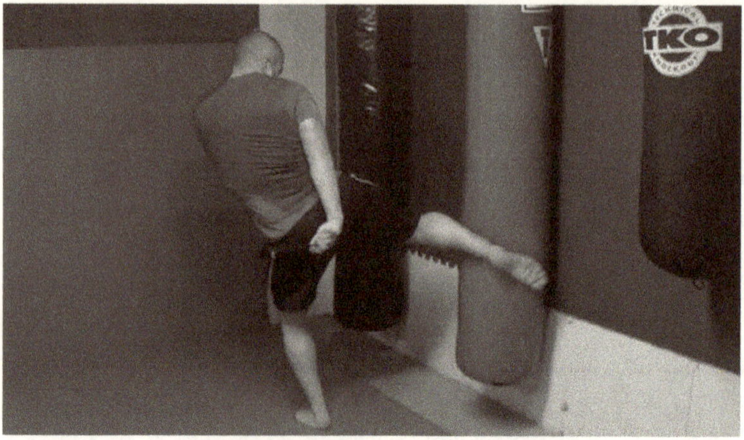

Figure 160: This time I have thrown the kick slightly higher. This kick would land on the mid to upper thigh of a person standing about 5"8". My shin would be placed solidly in the meat of their quadriceps (front of thigh). If you have never been kicked here, let me tell you that it hurts.

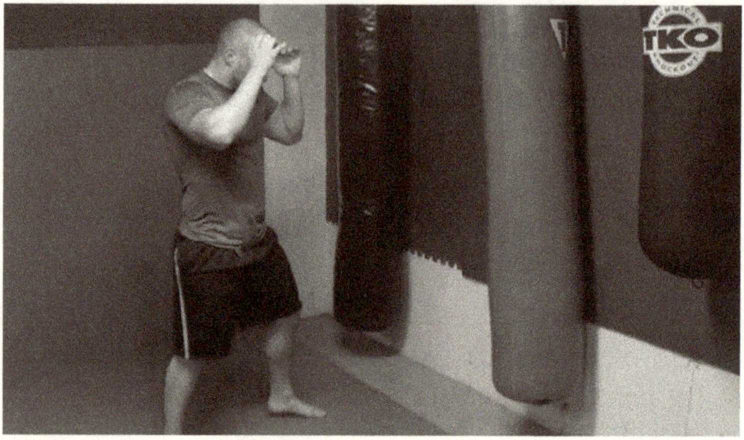

Figure 161: Return to the start position. Now you can throw a kick to the ribs of a person the same height as before.

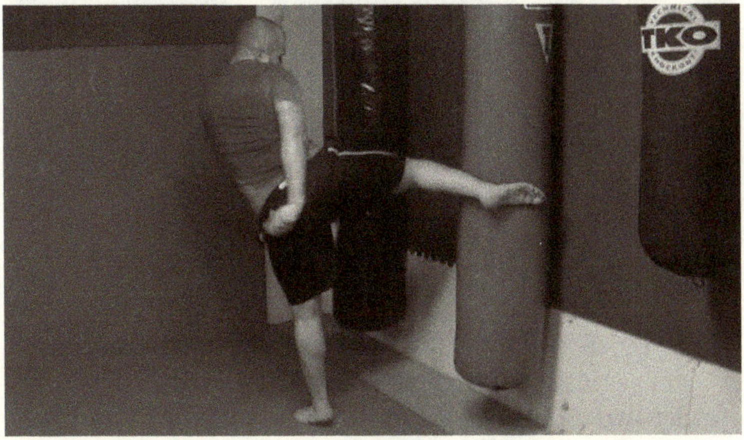

Figure 162: Now I have landed a kick that would be at rib level. This can knock the wind out of someone and break ribs. Remember that you are pivoting on your non-kicking foot and allowing your body to turn. However, you should not lose sight of your target. Your foot will hit what you are looking at.

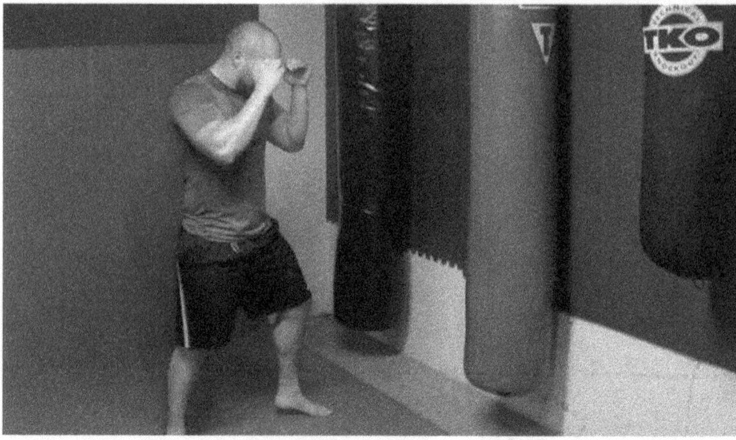

Figure 163: Return to the start position. You can now throw a kick to the neck/shoulder/head area. The path of the kick is the same.

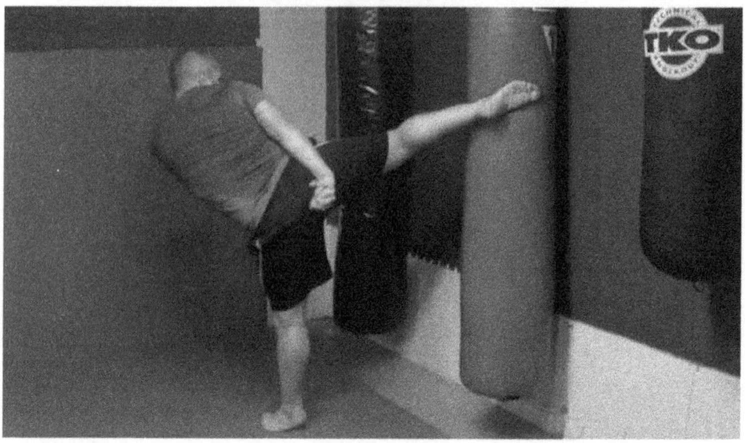

Figure 164: Notice that my leg has more extension this time. As kick height increases, it becomes less possibly to keep the bend in the leg and strike with the shin. As you near the end of your leg reach, extend fully and

strike the with the instep (area where the foot and ankle meet).

Kicks on a Suitcase Pad

A suit case pad is a common training item used in kick oriented martial arts. It is designed to absorb the impact of kicks in an efficient manner and to allow the striker to kick in a natural manner. Kicks follow the same pattern as normal when using the suitcase pad.

When using the suitcase pad, always know how hard the kicks are going to be. The person in control of the action should determine the strength of the kicks. Traditionally the pad holder determines the strength of the kick. He or she will call out various kicks in a predetermined strength. Regardless of who controls the training, the pad holder should always know how hard the kicks will be. In this manner, they can brace themselves for the kicks and training is safer.

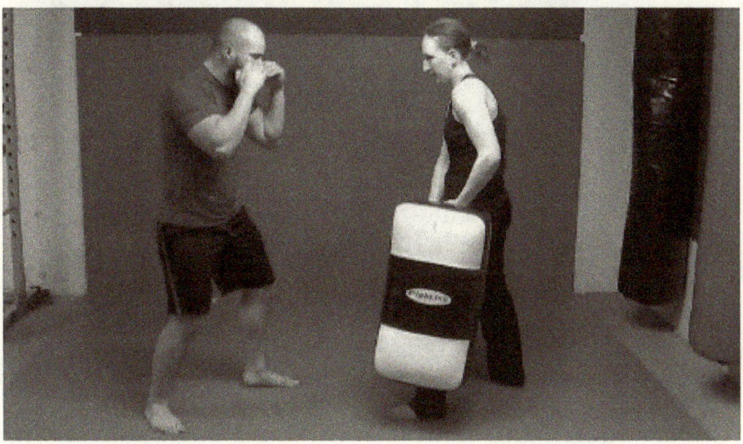

Figure 165: I set up for a round kick to knee level on the suitcase pad.

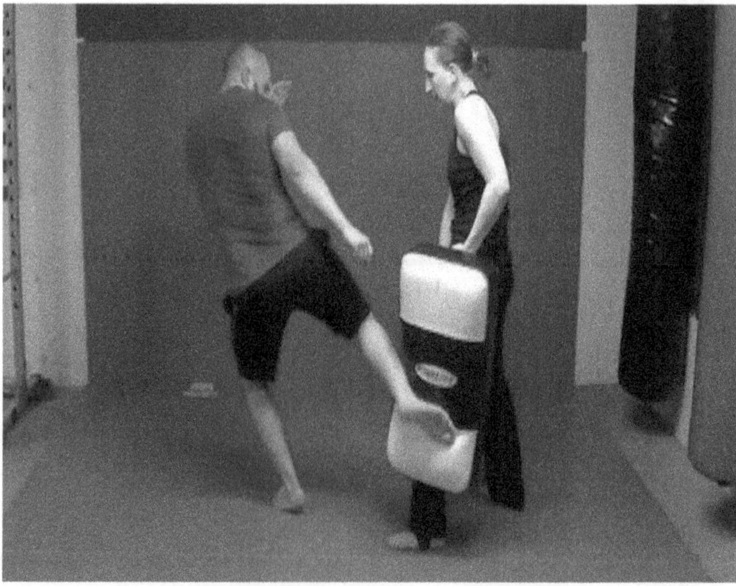

Figure 166: I throw the kick.

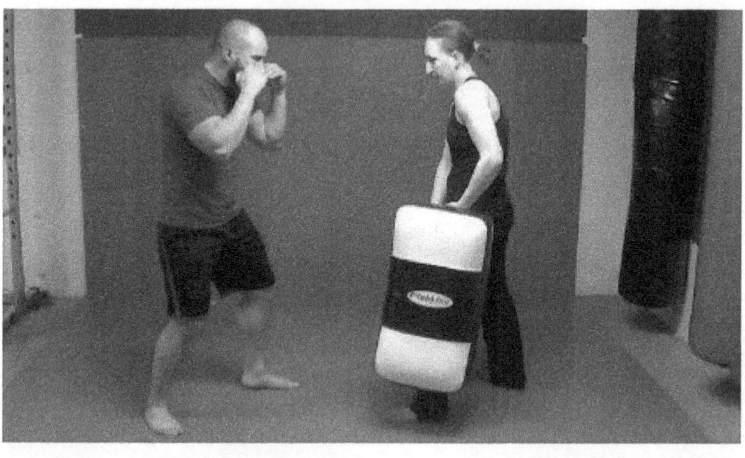

Figure 167: I reset and prepare to throw another kick.

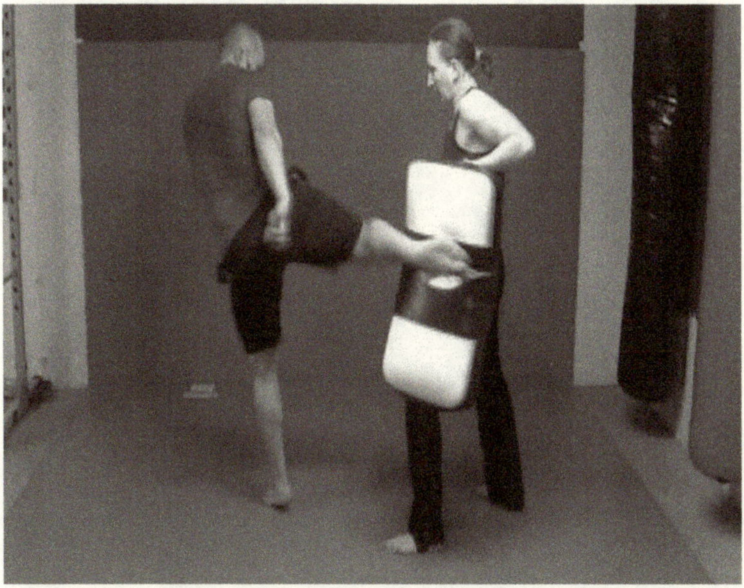

Figure 168: I throw a kick at about stomach level.

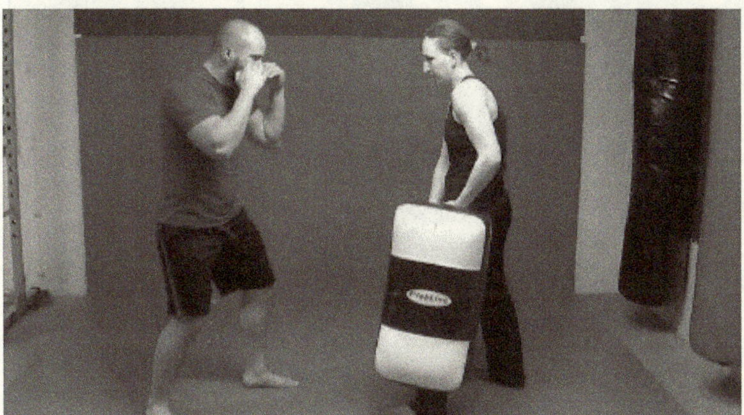

Figure 169: I reset again.

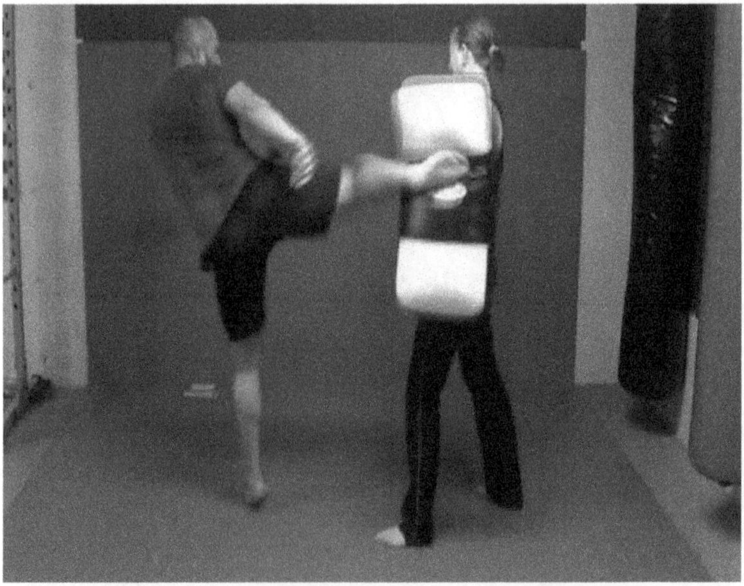

Figure 170: I throw a kick to the just below armpit level that would strike the ribs.

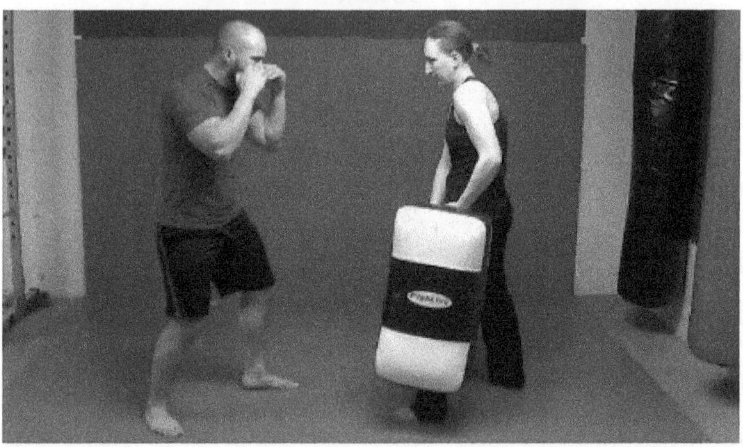

Figure 171: I reset again. You can practice like this with the suitcase pad. Single kicks, multiple kicks, front then rear, and other kicks can be thrown. Start simple and work up to advanced kicking.

The Front Round Kick

The front round kick can be accomplished in two ways. One is the switch kick. That will not be covered here. The other is a short round kick with the front leg in standard stance. This is just simply known as the front round kick. It does not have the power of the rear kick or the switch kick. However, with practice it can be thrown much quicker and can still have knockout capability.

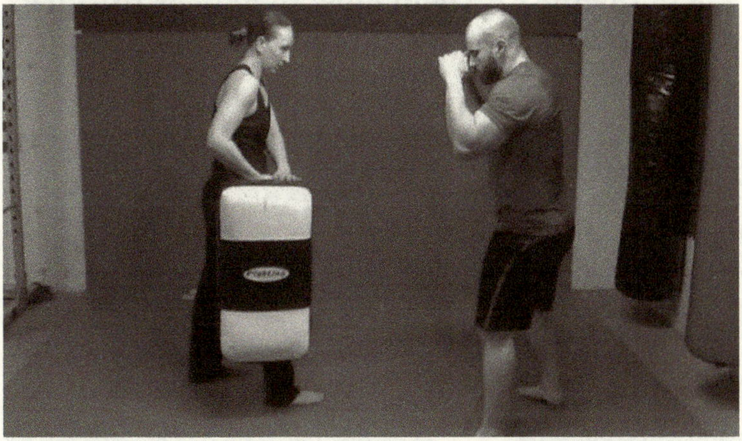

Figure 172: This kick can be delivered from the standard stance. You can also widen your stance to deliver this kick. That is what I have

done in this image. The wider stance allows a bit more torque, which will result in a stronger kick.

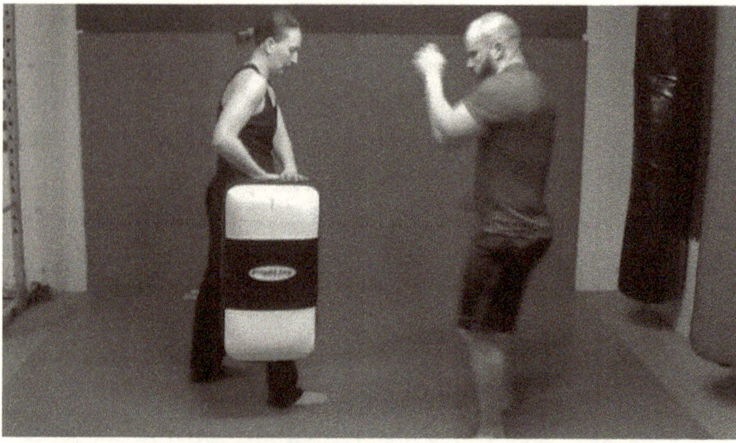

Figure 173: To deliver this kick I am sliding my rear foot forward just a bit which will allow me to torque and lean back to deliver the kick. You can try it without moving the foot forward.

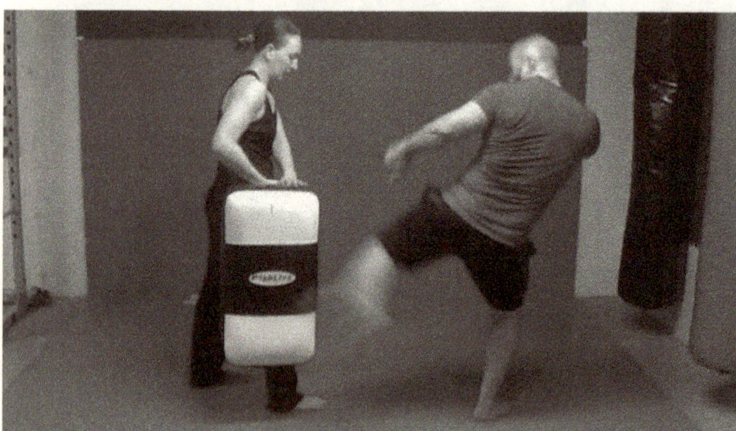

Figure 174: I pivot on my rear foot and begin the lean back. My kicking leg comes up and follows a small half-circle motion, similar to the rear round kick.

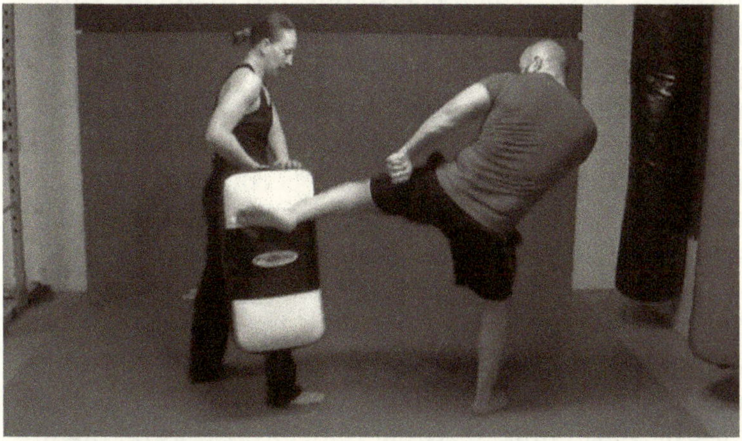

Figure 175: In this image, I have delivered a blow to the top of the thigh area.

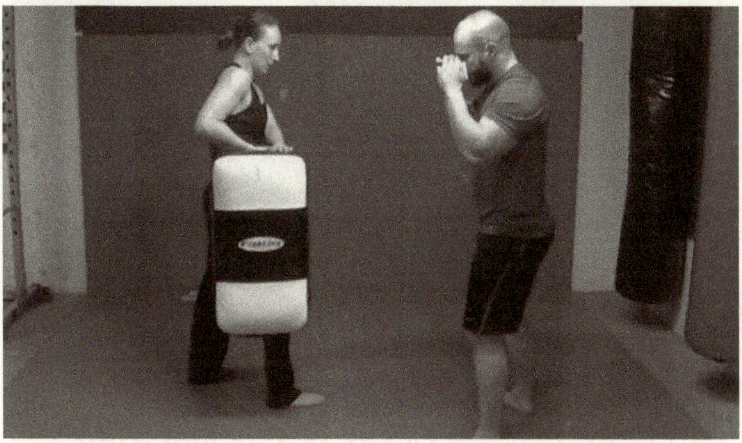

Figure 176: I return to start position.

Blocking Kicks

Blocking kicks, which is also referred to as checking kicks, is an essential defensive maneuver. More than punches, kicks hold damaging power. The power potential for the legs is far greater than that for the upper body. A person who takes too many kicks to the knee could find themselves with permanent knee damage. The same can be said for kicks to the thigh, or any other area for the matter.

When a person checks a low kick, they block the kick using their shin or the meat around the side of shin that make up part of the calf muscle. While taking the kick here will hurt, it will not hurt as bad as taking it on the knee or the thigh.

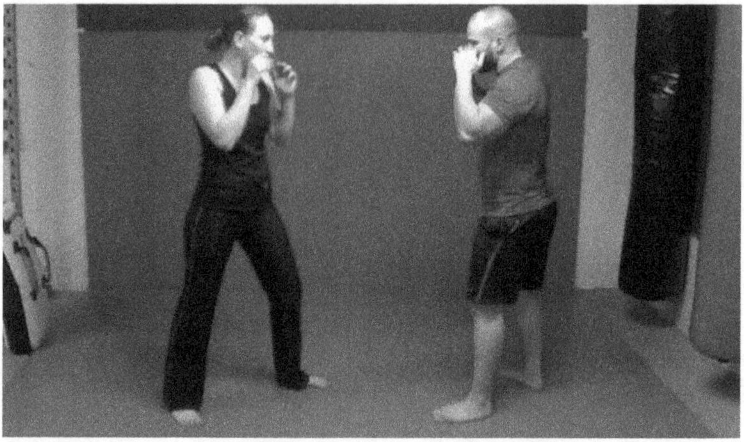

Figure 177: A kick can be blocked from essentially any stance.

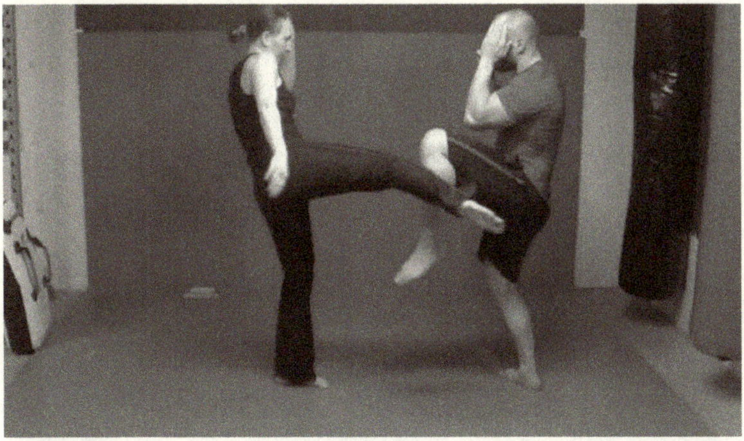

Figure 178: For best protection, it is ideal to block at the top and the bottom. In this image, you can see I am protecting my head with my hand and have lifted my leg to block the low kick. The reason for blocking top and bottom is to avoid shots to both locations. Clever fighters will fake a few kicks to one area, setting the defender to block this area, then throw one to the unblocked area.

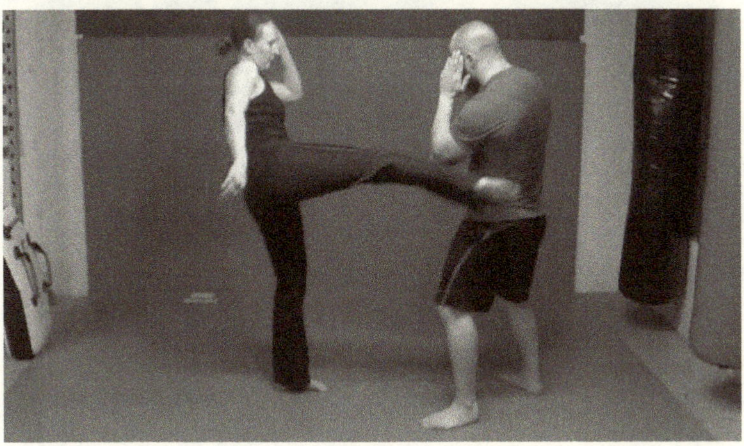

Figure 179: You can block singular areas. In this image, I am pulling my elbow to my side to defend against a rib strike.

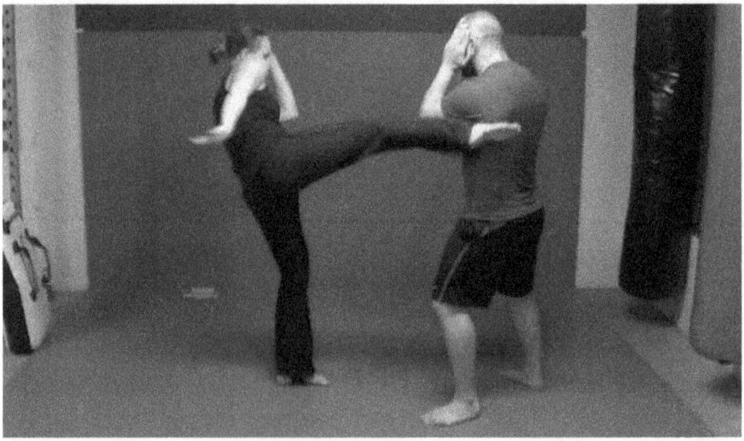

Figure 180: I use my elbow again here, this time to avoid a slightly higher kick.

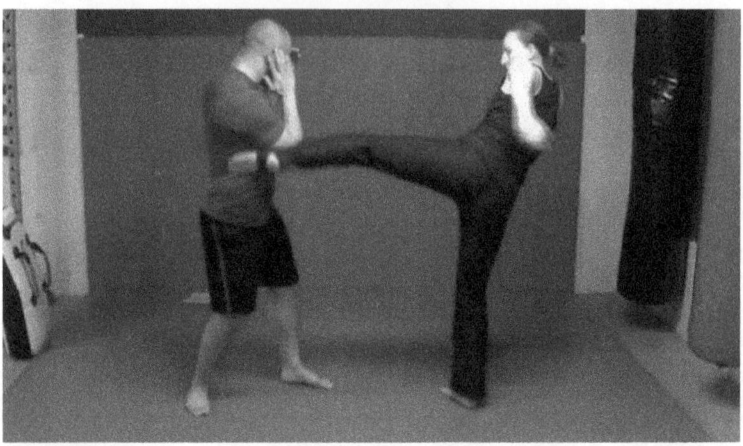

Figure 181: Here, I am blocking with my elbow on the opposite side.

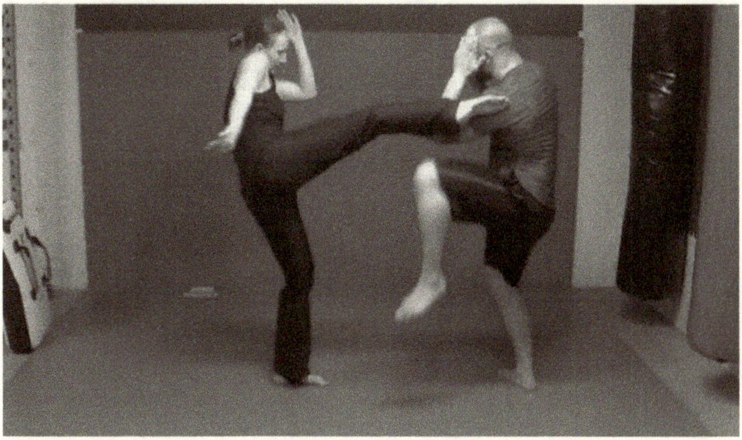

Figure 182: My partner in this image has not yet gained the flexibility to throw a high kick. However, she has thrown one to the shoulder and I am using a high block that would defend against a high kick.

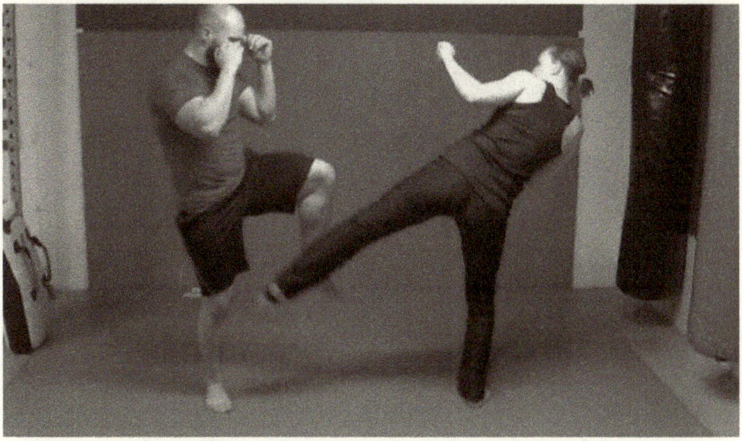

Figure 183: In this image, I am blocking against a knee level strike. I am not shielding against a high kick, although my hands are high as they always should be.

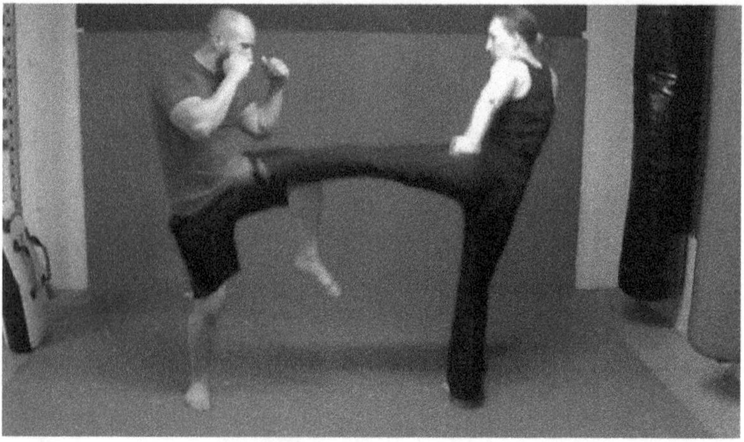

Figure 184: The same thing is happening here, except the opponent's kick would hit my stomach. Notice how I am using my knee in this image to block and in the last image I used the inside area of the shin/calf.

Chapter 6: Putting It Together

Once you have learned the individual moves you can start to chain together combos. You have already been introduced to some simple combos, the 1-2, and the #6 combo. You can build punch combos by working sections of the #6, mixing up punches, etc. The next series of images will show you how to mix punches with elbows and mix upper body strikes with lower body strikes. This will not be all inclusive of the number and pattern of combos available.

There are a finite number of combos available in martial arts standup striking. However, there are so many that the number may seem endless. This manual will cover but a few. Play around with combinations, experiment. The general rule of thumb is that combos should alternate sides. For example, you throw the jab in front of the cross. The reason for this is that the jab loads up the cross. The cross loads up the front hook and the front hook loads up the rear hook. Basically, when you throw a strike from one side you torque the other side and load up a shot from that side. Put combos together using this idea.

Now, combos can be thrown on the same side, but there is not wind up and this can take more skill. An example of a combo of the same side is the jab followed by the front hook. They both flow of the front hand. Now as mentioned this take more skill and practice. Start with alternating before moving on to same side strikes.

Another idea to follow is keeping it simple. I am all for fancy strikes and combos. I love Anthony Pettis style off the wall kicks and what not. That is actually a kick I have worked on for fun. However, being fancy may not be the best way to land strikes, especially outside of the ring where there are no rules. This is especially true if you are not as experienced with these moves. Anthony Pettis, and all other high-level fighters, have spent a great deal of time perfecting moves. With time, you can too, but in the beginning, keep it simple. Chain together simple punch, kick, knee, and elbow combos.

The following combos are examples you can start with. They are done in shadow boxing practice. This allows you to get the technique down and to learn to follow though. All of these combos can be practices on a heavy bag, suitcase pad, Thai pad, or focus mitts (each combo to their appropriate training item).

Combo 1: jab, cross, front uppercut, rear round kick

Combo 2: high rear kick, high rear kick, low rear kick (special combo)

Combo 3: cross, front uppercut, rear high kick

Jab, Cross, Front Uppercut, Rear Round Kick

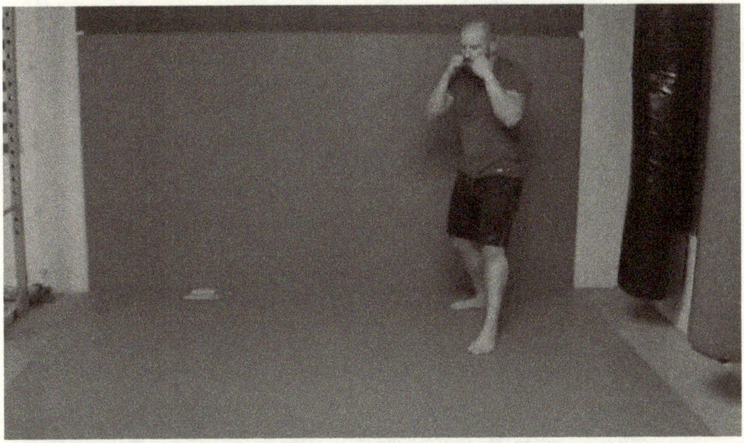

Figure 185: Start in stance.

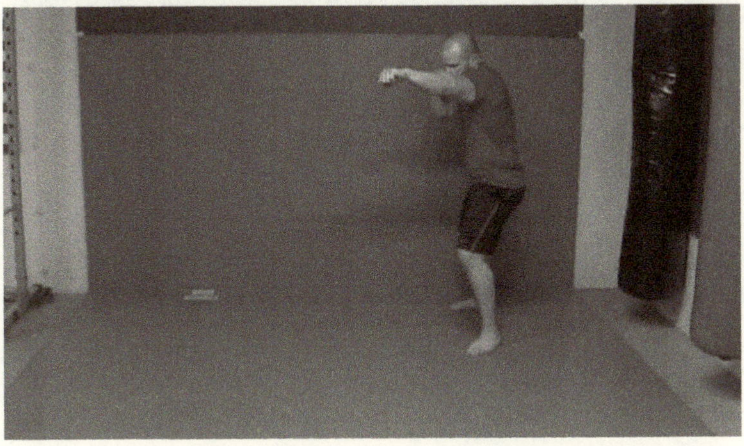

Figure 186: Throw the jab.

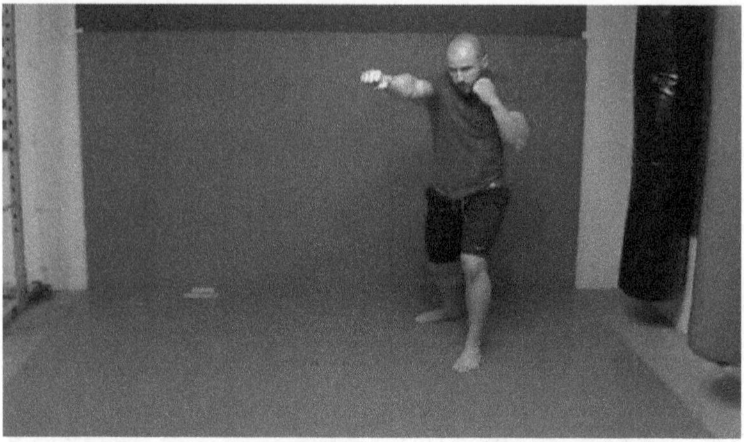

Figure 187: Throw the cross.

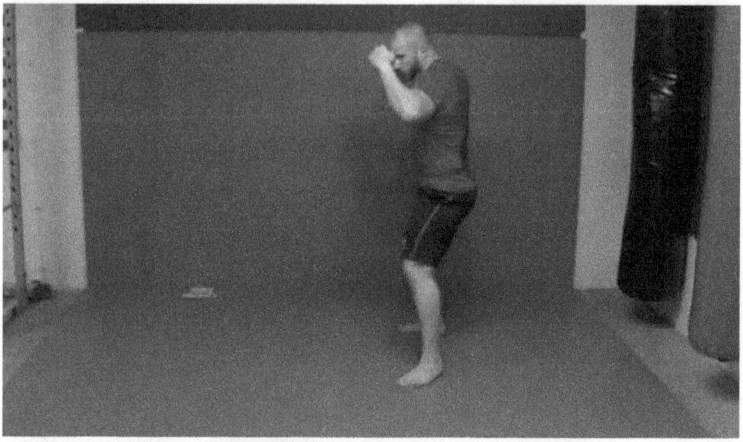

Figure 188: Throw the uppercut.

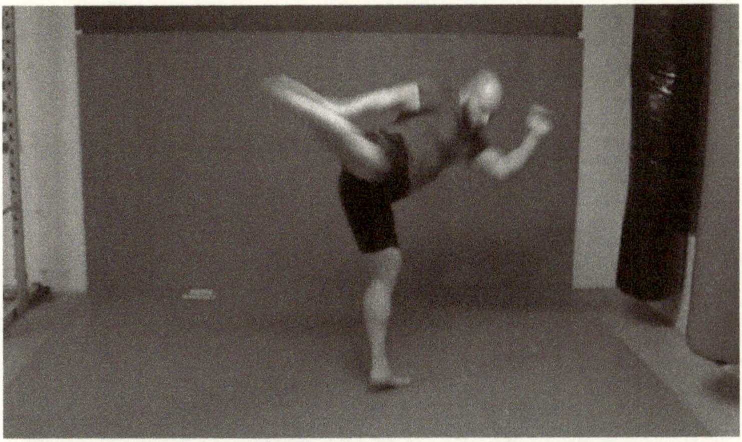

Figure 189: Throw the rear round kick.

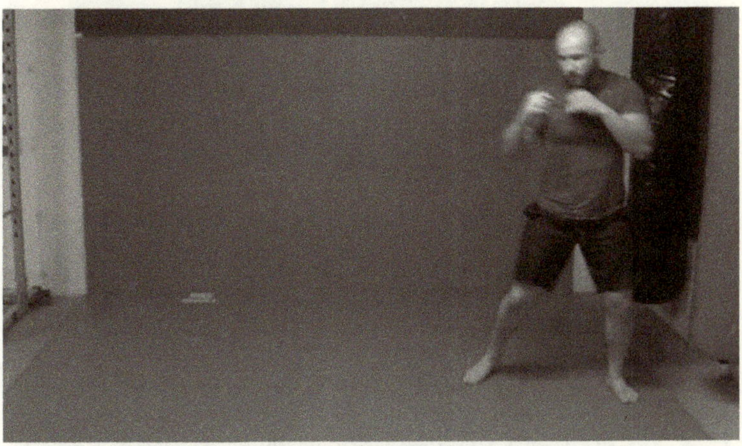

Figure 190: Follow thorough.

High Rear Kick, High Rear Kick, Low Rear Kick

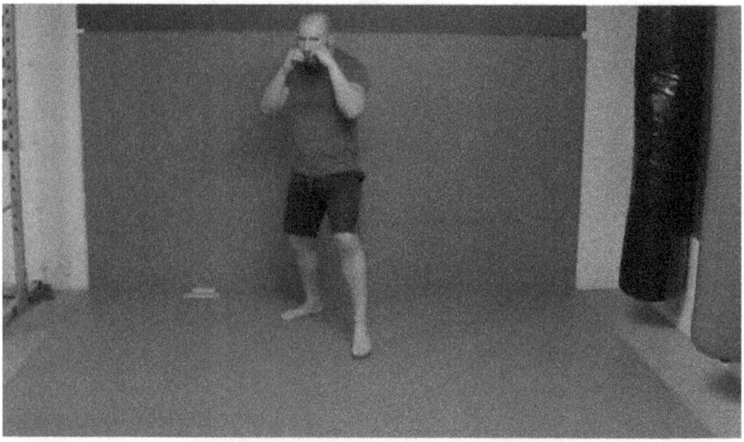

Figure 191: This combination is designed to teach you to follow through with the round kick.

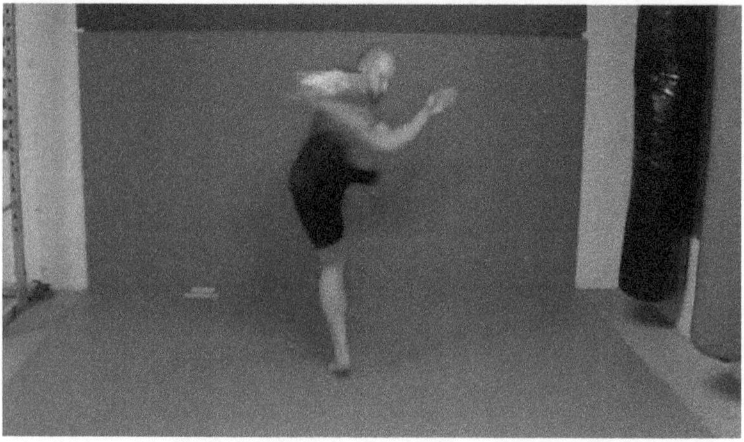

Figure 192: Throw a high round kick. If you can throw it at head level, then do so. If not, throw it as high as you can safely reach.

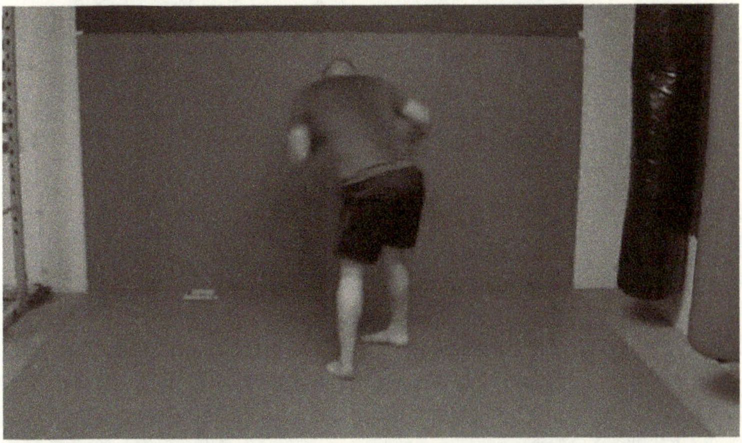

Figure 193: Follow through. This image shows me spinning out of the "missed" kick.

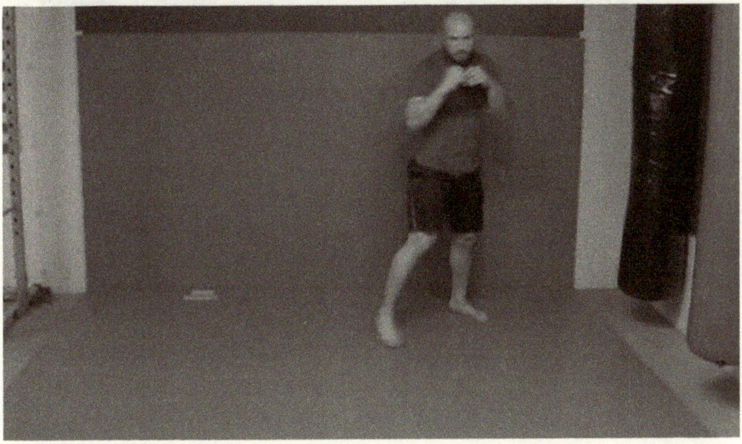

Figure 194: I have spun out of the kick and am in a southpaw stance.

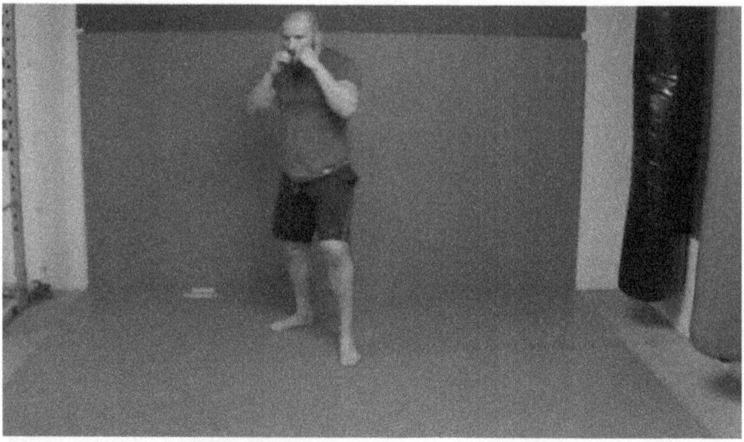

Figure 195: I return to my orthodox stance and prepare for the next kick.

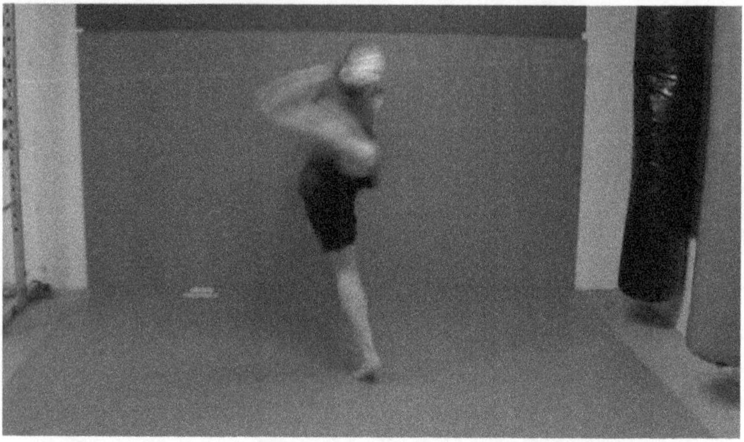

Figure 196: I throw the high kick again.

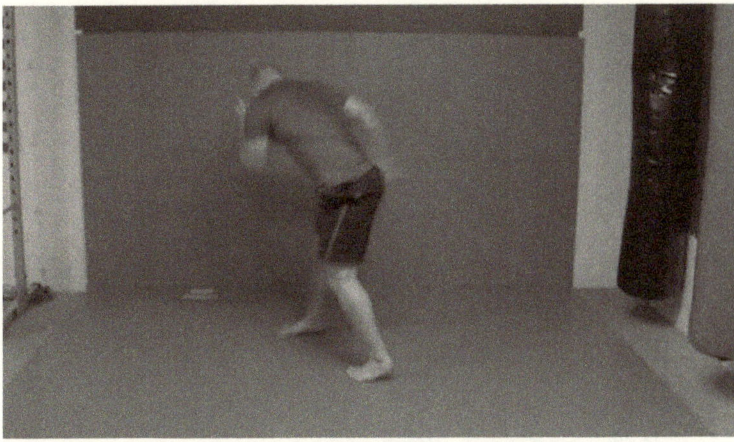

Figure 197: I spin through...

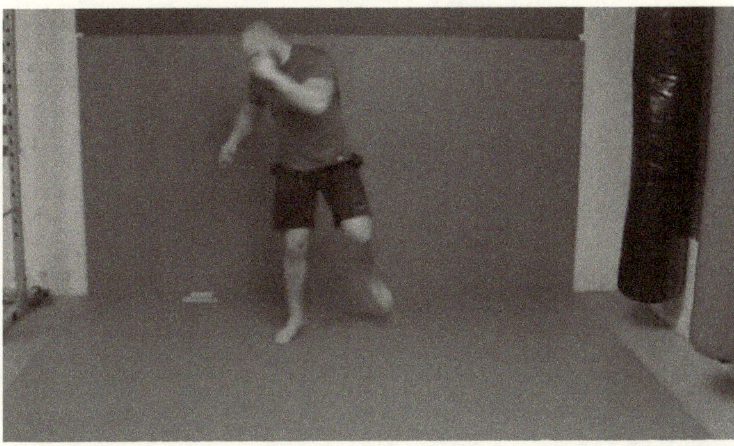

Figure 198: Allowing my body to follow the natural spin path.

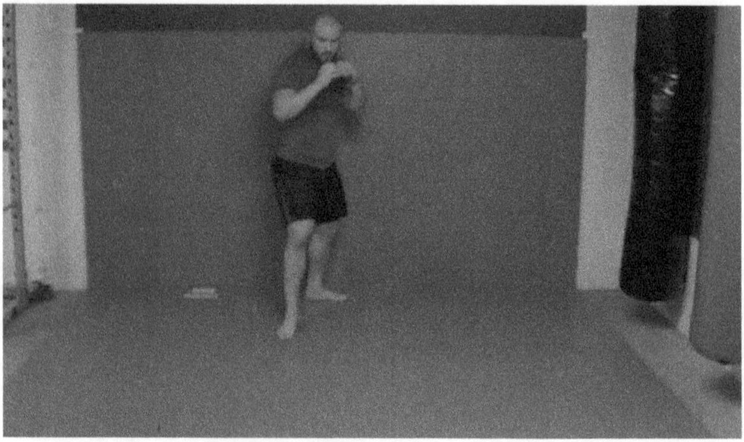

Figure 199: I land in the southpaw stance.

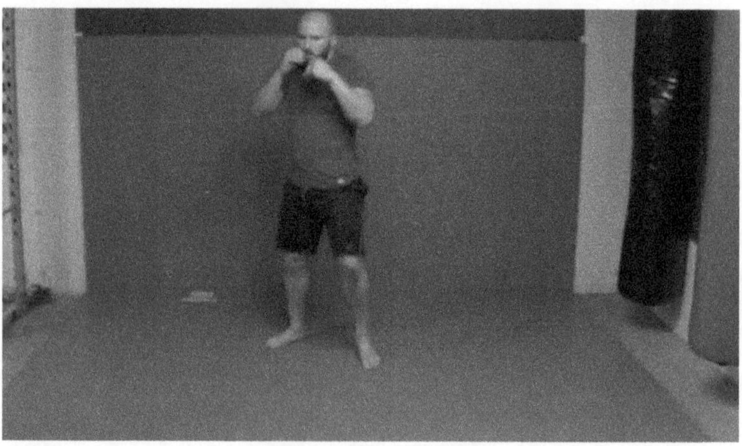

Figure 200: I return to my orthodox stance.

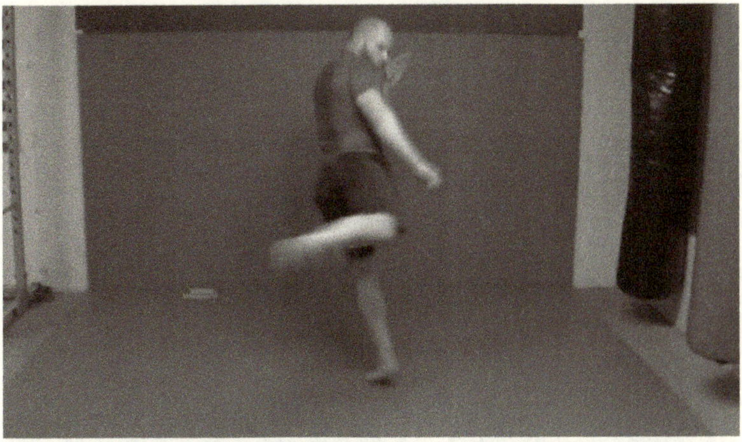

Figure 201: I quickly reset and throw the low kick.

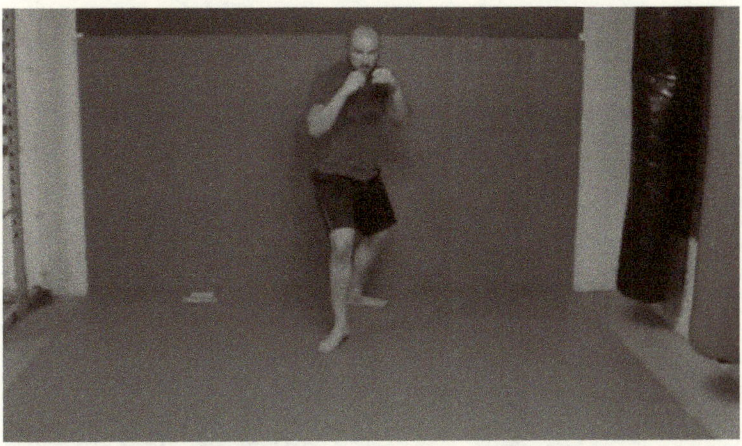

Figure 202: I follow through and land in the southpaw stance. This is a great way to learn to follow through. When performed on a heavy bag or suitcase pad it is great for generating speed and leg dexterity.

Cross, Front Uppercut, Rear High Kick

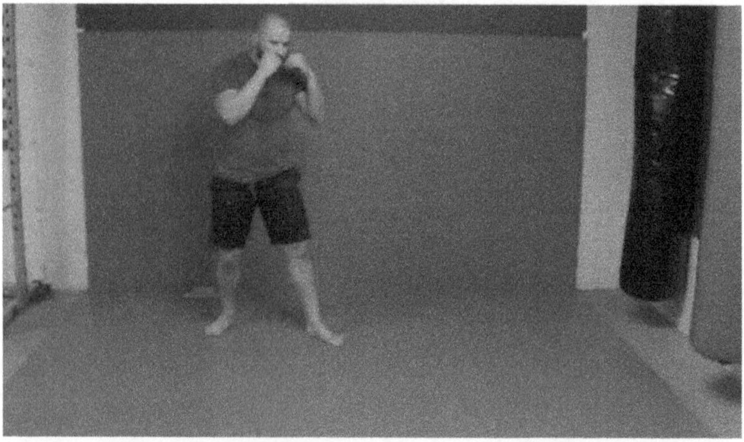

Figure 203: Start from your basic stance.

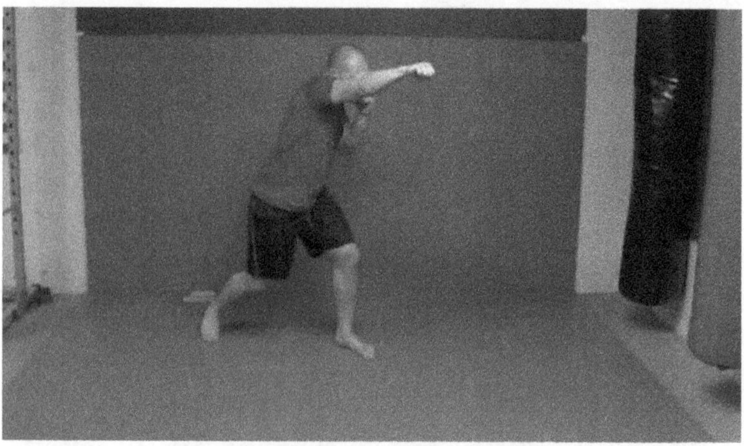

Figure 204: Throw the cross to the face.

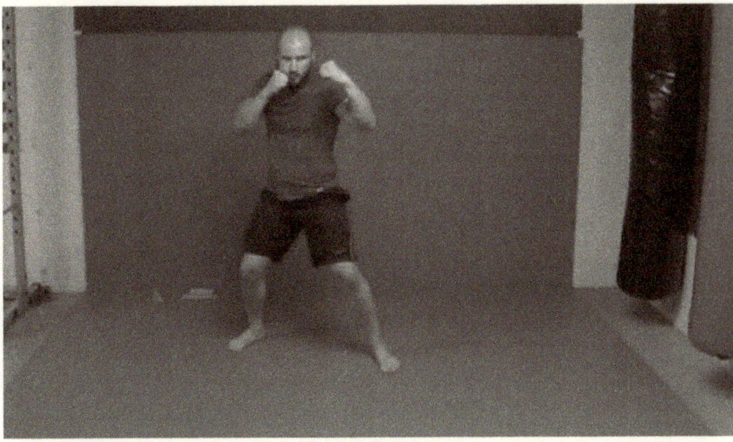

Figure 205: Throw the uppercut to the chin.

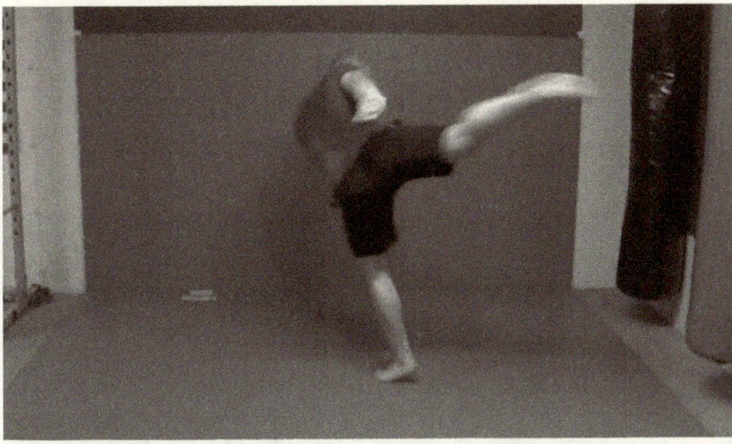

Figure 206: Throw the high kick.

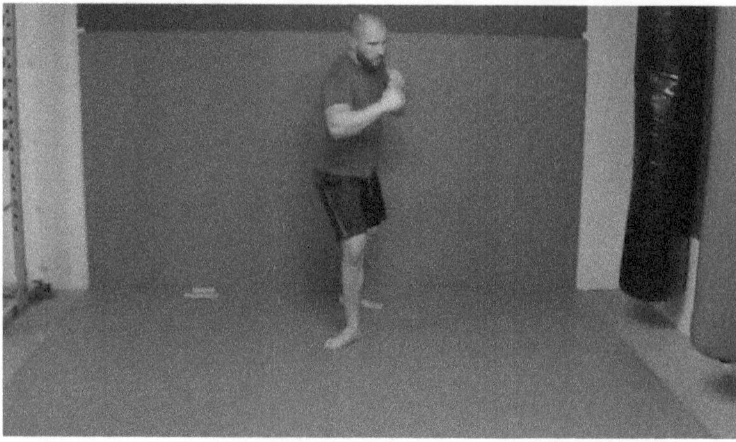

Figure 207: Follow through.

Cross, Front Uppercut, Rear Low Kick

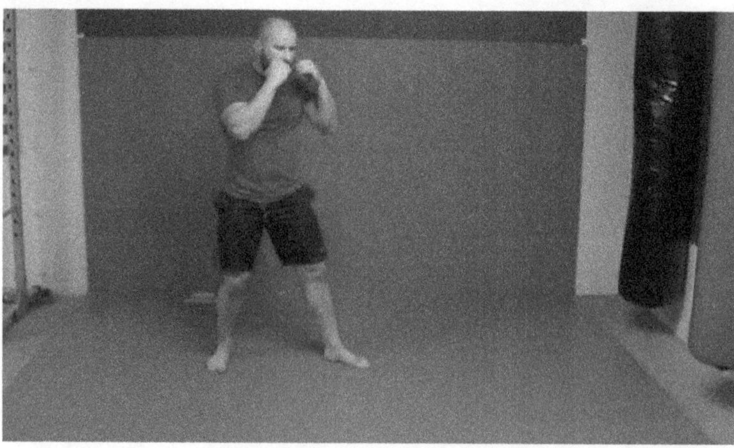

Figure 208: Start in your standard stance.

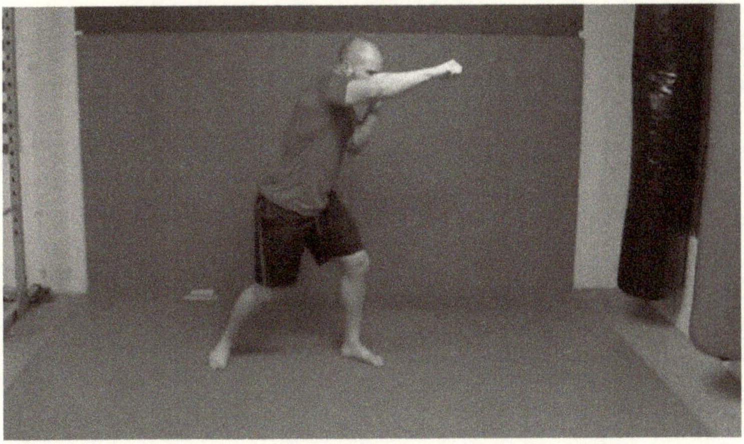

Figure 209: Throw the cross.

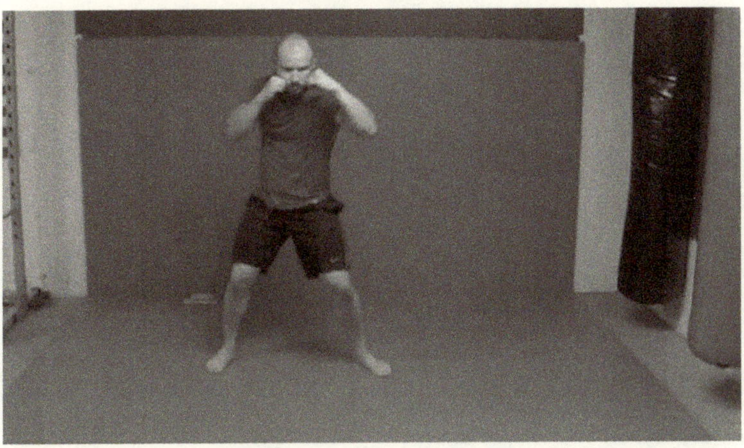

Figure 210: Throw the uppercut.

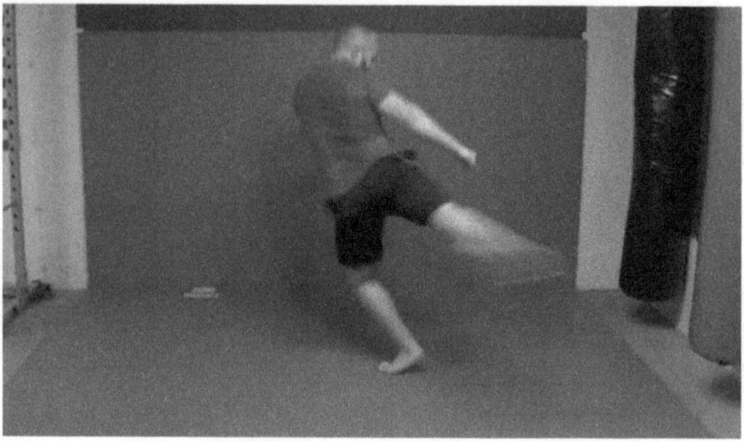

Figure 211:Throw the low kick.

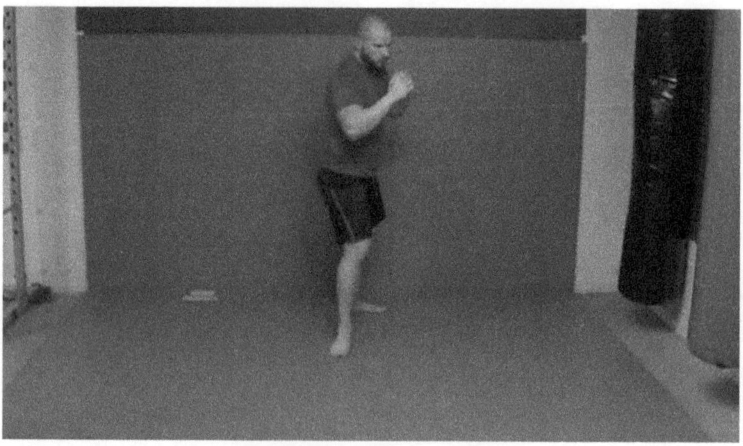

Figure 212: Follow through.

Jab, Cross, Front Elbow, Rear Elbow

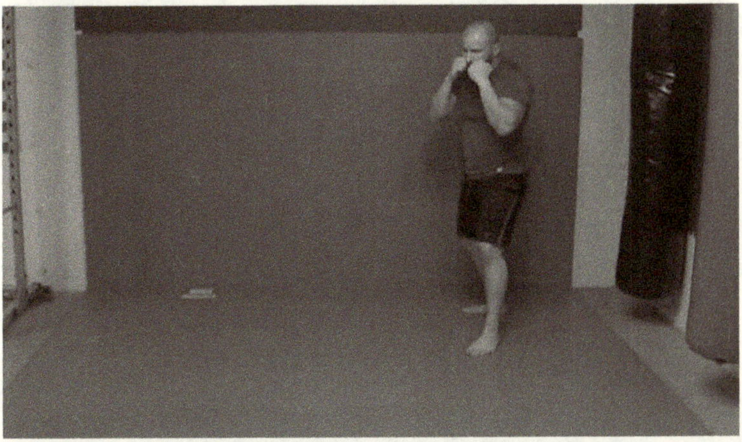

Figure 213: Start in stance.

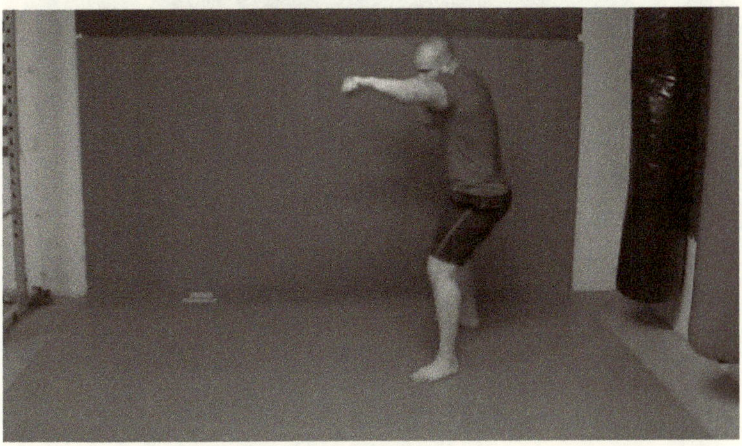

Figure 214: Throw the jab.

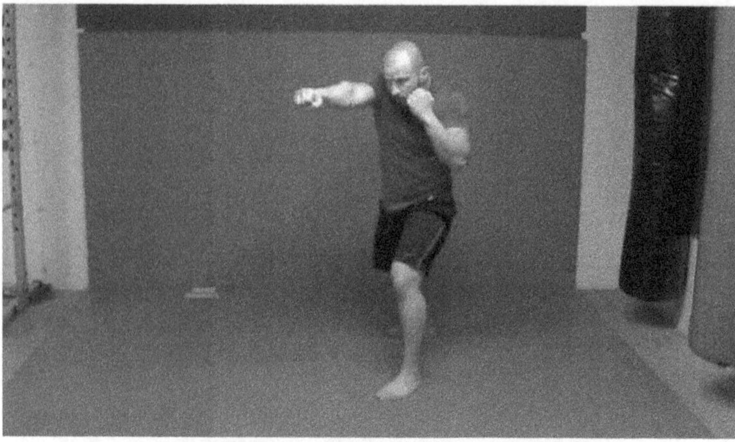

Figure 215: Throw the cross.

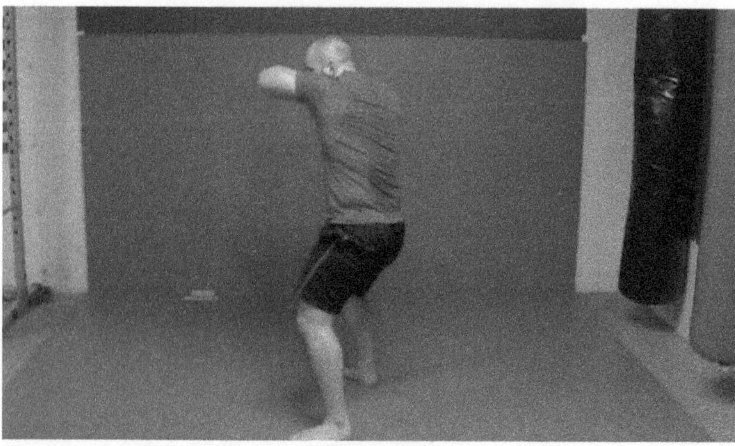

Figure 216: Throw the front elbow.

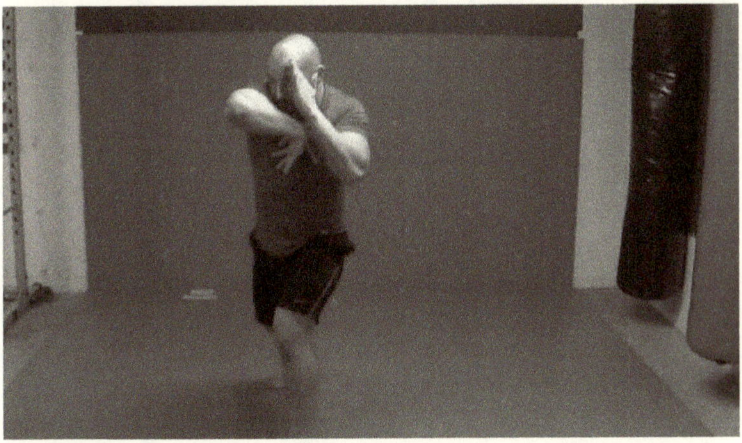

Figure 217: Throw the rear elbow. This combo is good if you are closing distance on an opponent.

I have a few final thoughts on shadow boxing. In these images, you will notice that I sometimes look toward my imaginary target and other times I look down. There is a reason for doing both. Whenever you are face to face with someone in a fight, you want to keep your eyes on the target. This allows you to see what they are doing in order to attack and defend properly.

Now, the reason I look down during some of the shadow boxing is to get a feel for the placement. I like to throw the punches and feel where they should be without seeing them. Sometimes I will throw the punch and stop it at the end of the strike. I will the look up to see if it is in proper form. This is kind of a personal form check. Sometimes I even close my eyes and just feel the movement. I have even applied this concept to grappling. I have practiced blind grappling, which is grappling while wearing a blindfold, to test how programmed moves are. This is not for everyone.

Use it if you feel comfortable and only after you have a solid understanding for the moves.

Conclusion: What's Next?

The preceding was a basic introduction to kickboxing, and (by default) boxing. It is meant to give you an idea of proper stance, movement, defense, and striking. It is not meant to teach you how to beat people up or be a bully. It is designed to teach you a form of self-defense and a way to stay fit. It is not meant to give you a cocky feeling so that you can act like a jerk. It is meant to build your confidence.

Moving forward you will need to practice quite a bit to get these techniques down. Once you do, you will have a well-rounded standup striking skill set. Make your training fun. If you do this, you are more likely to stick with it. One thing that can make training fun is to find a training partner who wants to learn with you but does not bring ego to training. Training needs to be cooperative and ego can get in the way of this.

Another way to make training fun is to avoid monotonous training. When I first started, I spent countless hours doing bag work and it was terrible. Did it help me learn? Well yeah, but once my training was mixed up I found it more enjoyable.

Here are some ideas for how to approach training:

- It is not an all effort all the time. Hitting the bag or training pads with 100% power every time will only wear you out and is not the best way to learn technique. Nice and easy is the way to go. The power will come.
- Do no more than one hour of training at a time, especially when training alone. If you have a

partner this time can increase because both of you will be doing the work. However, you should still ease into it.

- Organize your workouts in rounds. A stopwatch or timer will work for this purpose. iPods, Android devices, and other portable media devices usually have some sort of timer application. I personal use on from the iTunes store. It cost me a dollar. Set rounds at 3 or 5 minutes with a minute of rest between.
- Start your workouts with a solid warm-up such as vigorous footwork training and shadow boxing, a light run, or a dynamic warm-up. This will heat the muscles up and loosen them in the process. This will accelerate the heart and prep the body for work. Make this the first 2 – 4 rounds of your workout, depending on the round length. Follow the warm-up with some light pad or bag work and then work into heavy work. Use the last few rounds of your workout as a cool down. Do some shadow boxing or some footwork. End the workout with stretching.

That is all. You are ready to get to it. Be respectful of yourself and training partners. This leads to better training relationships and better results. Have fun and always train safe.

About the Expert

Nathan DeMetz is a personal trainer from Indiana. He has long been an avid fitness enthusiast and became a martial arts practitioner in recent years. He has been weight lifting for 12 years and practicing martial arts for three. Nathan is a Certified Personal Trainer (CPT)/Certified Fitness Trainer (CFT) with the International Sports Sciences Association (ISSA). He is a Certified Fitness Kickboxing Instructor through the Kickboxing Fitness Institute.

Nathan is currently pursuing Sport Nutrition Certification through ISSA. Nathan had the opportunity to meet and learn from a USAPL state ranked power lifter, two NPC bodybuilding competitors, and other local, amateur, and competitive athletes. He is the owner/operator of Nathan DeMetz Personal Training and the associated website, nathandemetz.com. Nathan has previously published "How To Jiu Jitsu For Beginners - Your-By-Step Guide To Jiu Jitsu For Beginners".

In 2010, Nathan started his martial arts journey with private boxing lessons from a local instructor before moving on to Muay Thai and jiu-jitsu. He is a white belt in jiu-jitsu and has 3 years of combined kickboxing experience. Nathan always looks to improve his skills through research, one-on-one conversation, and practical application.

Nathan competed in small-scale local competitions though he is not a competitive athlete in general. He simply enjoys the thrill of learning and practicing new forms of martial arts, as well as the rush he gets from weight lifting. Personal bests in weight training include a 500-lb. squat, 345-lb. bench, and a 530-lb. deadlift at a bodyweight between 185 lbs to 213 lbs.

Outside of athletics, Nathan is a family man and everyday guy. He has a 2-year Business degree that he has used in management and now uses as a self-employed contractor. He primarily provides Internet based services to online clients. His list of clients includes Google, Ask.com and eBay. He is married and has been with his wife, Grace, for almost 7 years. Nathan has a daughter from a previous relationship who will be sixteen this year.

Away from work and training, Nathan enjoys spending time with his wife and daughter. He also enjoys fat burgers with French fries and juicy steaks.

HowExpert publishes quick 'how to' guides on all topics from A to Z by everyday experts. Visit HowExpert.com to learn more.

Recommended Resources

- HowExpert.com – Quick 'How To' Guides on All Topics from A to Z by Everyday Experts.
- HowExpert.com/free – Free HowExpert Email Newsletter.
- HowExpert.com/books – HowExpert Books
- HowExpert.com/courses – HowExpert Courses
- HowExpert.com/clothing – HowExpert Clothing
- HowExpert.com/membership – HowExpert Membership Site
- HowExpert.com/affiliates – HowExpert Affiliate Program
- HowExpert.com/writers – Write About Your #1 Passion/Knowledge/Expertise & Become a HowExpert Author.
- HowExpert.com/resources – Additional HowExpert Recommended Resources
- YouTube.com/HowExpert – Subscribe to HowExpert YouTube.
- Instagram.com/HowExpert – Follow HowExpert on Instagram.
- Facebook.com/HowExpert – Follow HowExpert on Facebook.